THE IGNORAMUS SERIES 1

UNDERSTANDING THE SILENT KILLER DISEASES

BY DR. EUGENE C. UCHE

Published on CreateSpace.

ISBN-13: 978-1502548931

ISBN-10: 1502548933

Acknowledgement

I am forever grateful to God who empowered me by his grace and has brought me this far, even when all odds were against me.

To my beautiful wife and kids, your overwhelming support was the right prescription when I needed comfort and strength; you are truly a blessing. I couldn't have asked for a better family.

To my adopted mother and boss, Mrs. Bonnie Triggs, thank you for being a mother when I truly needed one. God has promised that he will reward you with long healthy life and you shall eat the fruits of your labor.

To my mentor, Mr. Lenwood O'Neal, we are inseparable! Thank you so much for everything you taught me. I will forever be grateful.

DEDICATION

This book is dedicated to my beloved brother the late Dr. Stanley Uche, who was murdered in Nigeria (September 2010) while providing selfless services to the poverty trodden masses in Nigeria. To all the physicians and health workers who selflessly gave their life while caring for Ebola infected patients all over the African nations- Dr. Ameyo Stella Adadevoh (Nigeria-2014), Dr. Oliver Buck (Sierra Leone-2014), Dr. Sheik Humar Khan (Sierra Leone-2014) and Dr. Samuel Brisbane (Liberia-2014) and many others; your sacrifices to humanity, especially those who could not afford to defend themselves from silent killer diseases will never be forgotten.

CONTENTS

CHAPTER 1

INTRODUCTION

The perceptions of diseases are quite different in developing countries compared to the developed nations. People's belief and perception of health has an impact on the nation's public health initiative, implementation, preventions and outcome. The differences in perception and approach in this case has less to do with technological modernization, and more to do with culture and lack of basic disease etiology.

For example, it was not until recently that the disease "sleeping sickness" otherwise known as African Trypanosomiasis-a progressive fetal neurological disease, was accepted as an illness in most parts of the country. This disease literally rendered most parts of many African nations lifeless for both human and domestic animals. The problem here was not that the people embraced the devastation caused by this disease; rather, the lack of knowledge of symptoms of the disease and that it is not a witch attack made it difficult for the people to seek help in the right places.

In fact, in some parts of the developing world, people believe that disease outbreak is a punishment from a supernatural deity and this belief has led to the delay in searching for the right cures or practices and has helped in spreading the disease. For few who are eager to seek answers, culture and traditional belief (most of their theory has no basis) provides cruel non-researched based myths packaged like truth. God knows how many lives will be negatively impacted before culture will changes.

August 4, 1990, in Nigeria, my father's big brother uncle James was admitted to the hospital for abdominal cramps, diarrhea, and vomiting. According to his wife, the symptoms started a couple of days earlier in the middle of the night and by early morning the symptoms increased to dizziness, tearing in the eyes and excessive salivation. By this time, he was self-medicating himself with local herbs hoping everything will be alright. By the sunset that evening, he started experiencing mental confusion, partial loss of speech and vision, muscle weakness, difficulty swallowing, dry mouth, muscle paralysis from the head down through the body. While in the hospital, the doctor came in and reassured my uncle once again that he will be alright and informed him that he is suffering from bacterial infection *botulism.* My uncle asked the doctor what the source of the bacteria could be and the doctor innocently said, "food poisoning!"

Well, a few days later my uncle was discharged from the hospital. About 6 days after he was discharged, the traditional ruler of our town summoned all the family members and declared that my uncle's wife will be excommunicated from the village for an alleged attempt to kill her husband "my uncle." At the beginning it was like a joke but little did I know that it was my uncle who reported his wife to the traditional ruler. About an hour later after the king passed his judgment, the youth of my village stormed the compound and literally dragged the woman (my uncle's wife back to her family). It was very humiliating and as a very young boy I could not help her. Fifteen years later, I can still remember the look in her face pleading *"Onwekwa ihemere"* –I am innocent!

She was sent home to her family for 11 years just because the word "food poisoning" was mentioned and my uncle's belief that if he was poisoned through food, then, his wife must be his prime suspect.

Unfortunately, the people (the king, my uncle and other family members) were ignorant of common causes of food poisoning. Although food poisoning is an illness caused by eating or drinking contaminated food; it does not mean that someone actually intentionally poisoned him. One can get food poisoning by eating food contaminated by harmful organisms, such as bacteria, parasites, and viruses.

In Africa, our environmental pollution is a very big public health concern. In fact people buy Mangoes and other fruits and vegetables on the road with little or no effort to clean it. They just wipe the dirt off and eat it. There are several possibilities and sources of food poisoning especially for someone living in a developing country, but that lady suffered 11 years of shame and humiliation, and 15 years of marriage placed on hold for a crime she did not commit.

In South Africa, a country long-sickened by the level of sexual violence, a shocking series of child rapes was reported in 2002- (IRIN, 2002). In 2011, Betty Makoni in her documentary movie *Tapestries of Hope* exposed the "Virgin Cleansing Myth" which is another unspeakable crime to humanity. According to the news magazine "The Telegraph," as many as ten girls are raped every day. As many as 3,600 girls in Zimbabwe each year may be contracting HIV/AIDS after being raped. The Virgin Cleansing Myth theory believes and accepts the myth that sex with a virgin cleanses one of HIV/AIDS. Cases were reported in which a one-day-old infant girl was raped by six men in a remote part of rural South Africa just because someone believed that this cruel act is a cure for HIV/AIDS.

In 2002 in South Africa, more than 67,000 cases of rape and sexual assaults against children were reported. The most terrifying part of this story is that the rapists were all HIV positive men looking for possible cure for the disease. Some of the victims died from their injuries, while others contracted HIV.

Ignoramus on its own is a disease- a silent killer disease.

In different parts of developing countries, baseless conspiracy theorists have acted ignorantly against public health initiative put together to improve the health of the citizens. For example, in the summer of 2003, Muslim clerics and disgruntled northern politicians engaged in a year-long ban on a polio vaccinations initiative in the Northern part of Nigeria, claiming that the drugs were a Western ploy to spread HIV and sterilize Muslim girls. This abrupt halt in vaccination sparked a rash of new infections, and the virus jumped to about a dozen other countries in the region.

One of the public health recommendations for preventing HIV/AIDS infection is the use of Condom during sexual intercourse. Meanwhile, Time online magazine reported that, "*One strong belief held by a number of Africans is that the West wants to control the population growth of Africa, and that the West is trying to do this by convincing Africans to use condoms. The West is encouraging African nations to use condoms as protection against AIDS, but many Africans believe that this is just a ploy to curb reproduction*"

The 2007 world health report, "A Safer Future', claimed that today's highly mobile, interdependent and interconnected world provides a myriad of opportunities for the rapid spread of diseases..." There is no doubt that the rate of the spread of infectious diseases is much faster now than ever before. Between the months of March to July 2014, Ebola virus spread from Guinea to Liberia to Sierra Leone to Nigeria killing more than 700 people and infecting more than 1300.

Unfortunately, the so-called world interconnectedness failed to provide, in most cases, corresponding capability for the people in the rural part of the developing countries to identify those diseases, especially at the onset stages.

A few years ago, WHO health report "The health of the people" acknowledged the severity of the health crisis faced by African nations and other developing countries. About 738 million African residents faced a dramatic health crisis according to the report. The report also suggested that international support is highly needed in order to diffuse this time bomb.

Meanwhile, there have been undeniable efforts by the World Health Organization and other agencies to help reduce disease epidemics in different parts of the developing nations; however, ignorance has successfully undermined these efforts. The good news remains that, Ignoramus as a disease has just one active prescription - knowledge. This book is an antidote to the disease of public health "ignoramus" among many people in Africa and other parts of the developing world.

The depth of knowledge provided in this book offers hope and will defeat hopelessness, and literally put the reader in the driver's seat where public health is concerned; arm our people to battle and defeat the silent killer diseases. While it is the responsibility of every government to provide basic healthcare system for their citizenry, being healthy is the sole responsibility of the citizenry. The main purpose of this book is to equip the reader with the information necessary to become and remain healthy; differentiate between diseases infection and witchcraft attack.

According to "The Health of the People", although HIV/AIDS remains the leading cause of death for adults, more and more persons are receiving life-saving treatment. The number of HIV-positive people on antiretroviral medicines increased eight-fold, from 100,000 in December 2003 to 810,000 in December 2005. If you recall, this was not the case a few years ago. In fact, study shows that lack of basic knowledge of symptoms of this disease resulted in the spread of HIV/AIDS in Africa and many other developing countries. There were different conspiracy theories regarding the etiology of the virus. The unfortunate thing then was that most of the practices that claimed to heal HIV/AIDS patients actually fueled the incidence rate of HIV/AIDS.

For example, in some parts of Africa, it was reported that some traditional beliefs forced widows to have sex with their dead spouse's corps to ensure the spirit of the dead spouse rests in peace. Unfortunately, a majority of this cruel traditional belief is dormant among the poor and underprivileged women. Hold on now; was there any autopsy report to determine the cause of death of the spouse? Could it be that the husband died of one of the notorious silent killer diseases such as HIV/AIDS, with the virus still breathing in the corpse's semen, the wife just got baptized with the disease.

Nelson Mandela, former South African president (bless his memories), once stated that, "Education is such a powerful ammunition that can be used to change our world". According to John F. Kennedy, "The basic goal for aspiring for education shall be for the advancement of knowledge and disseminating truth". The search for truth has resulted in many unexplained and unproven theories. However, truth in its raw form is never tainted and when it is by human quest for knowledge or intentional deception, belief and cultural inhumanity, catastrophe is inevitable. Light has never failed as an antidote to darkness, so has knowledge and truth. It does not matter how thick the darkness, a single ray of light makes an enormous difference.

As an agent of social change, it is impossible for some of us to literally "just stand aside and look" while our prophets are being slaughtered (*Bob Marley*). Unfortunately, our world is so big that no one man can change it alone, but our collective effort – disseminating the truth - is our weapon of mass reconstruction.

Ignoramus has proven not to be an excuse. An African school of thought stated that, "what you don't know will not harm you". I wish that statement was true. Africa and most of the developing nations would have been the safest place to live in terms of quality of life and well-being. Disease (communicable and non-communicable) outbreaks in most parts of the world including Africa and its devastative nature have proven that ignorance cannot deliver you from the destructive hand of disease. Rather, knowledge has proven to be a progressive discovery of our ignorance.

Even one of the bestselling religious books (Bible) acknowledged the importance of education and knowledge and stated, *"How will they know except someone teaches them..." (Romans 10:14).* Could it be that one of the ways (if not the only way) we can change the state of public health in our nations is through education on disease etiology, prevention and control. How will they understand that disease or ill-health is not necessarily a punishment from a supernatural being or witchcraft except we educate them? Even if they are, education and knowledge have provided an alternative; most diseases can be prevented, controlled and even treated or eradicated. However, human beings have a major role to play in this game.

"Patients' health beliefs can have a profound impact on clinical care. They can impede preventive efforts, delay or complicate medical care and result in the use of folk remedies that can be beneficial or toxic. Culturally-based attitudes about seeking treatment and trusting traditional medicines and folk remedies are rooted in the core belief systems about illness causation"……Marcia Carteret, M. Ed.(date unknown)

As one travels from one region or nation of the world through another, you notice that there are varying cultural views on the relationship between public health and disease causation. For example, a physician in the United State or European countries through his medical training believes in the Germs theory of a common cold and flu influenza. A Babalawo (faith healers) in Africa believes that the common cold comes from an evil spirit. While the American or European physician believes in vaccination and hand hygiene as a remedy for prevention of common cold and flu, the African faith healer believes that the gods are demanding scarify. Until cultural ignoramuses are properly addressed, the actual disease causation will not be addressed.

This book is aimed to close the gap between what is known and what we believe; what we can see (through medical diagnosis) and what we assume. Silent killer diseases are real; you have to stop them before they stop you.

CHAPTER 2
WITCHCRAFT AND PUBLIC HEALTH

In attempt to describe the etiology of disease, two major systems have been developed by some schools of thought. The first is the personalistic system of disease etiology which believes that disease is as a result of supernatural being with special powers. The second system of belief is the naturalistic system; this system believes that a person's health is a factor of its environment. That means a healthy condition is attained when an equilibrium balance is reached between what is sane and insane; between your environment and the state of your environment.

The concept and attributing of disease to witchcraft varies from one region to another. Merriam-Webster's Collegiate Thesaurus defines Witchcraft as the use of sorcery or magic, communication with the devil or familiar, an irresistible influence or fascination. The dictionary associates witchcraft with words such as, bewitchery, bewitchment, conjuring, devilry, diablerie, enchantment, voodooism, magic, witchery and wizardry. The first known use of witchcraft was in the 12th century.

The origin of Witchcraft, and the argument whether witchcraft exists or not is beyond the scope of this book. Meanwhile, the cultural attributes of disease etiology to witchcraft and its impact on public health disease education, treatment and control remain in part the focus of this book. A 2009 Gallup poll face-to-face interview of 18,000 adults 15 years and older from18 sub-Sahara African countries: Burundi, Cameroon, Chad, Congo Kinshasa, Ghana, Ivory Coast, Kenya, Mali, Nigeria, Rwanda, Senegal, South Africa, Tanzania, Uganda, Zambia, and Zimbabwe; on whether they "believe in witchcraft" shows a disturbing degree of belief in witchcraft. About 55% of African respondents' reported that they believe in witchcraft or witchery culture.

Do you personally believe in witchcraft?

	Yes	No	Don't know/ Refused
Ivory Coast	95%	5%	0%
Senegal	80%	19%	2%
Ghana	77%	21%	2%
Mali	77%	23%	1%
Cameroon	76%	24%	0%
Congo (Kinshasa)	76%	24%	0%
Niger	75%	24%	0%
Malawi	72%	28%	0%
Chad	68%	31%	0%
Tanzania	64%	36%	0%
Zimbabwe	63%	37%	0%
Zambia	59%	41%	1%
AVERAGE	55%	43%	2%
South Africa	46%	54%	0%
Burundi	46%	55%	0%
Nigeria	45%	49%	5%
Kenya	26%	74%	0%
Rwanda	17%	83%	0%
Uganda	15%	85%	0%

Surveys conducted between April and December 2009

GALLUP

Another interesting but alarming part of this report is the demography of the respondents. The survey reported that the older and less educated the respondents were the more likely they were to believe in witchcraft than the younger and more educated respondents. Meanwhile, I am not ignorant of the educated fools among us; those whom despite their high level of education, still rely on voodoo and witch doctor to diagnose and treat health conditions when obvious symptoms of high blood pressure and glaucoma exist in their body.

Also, in terms of satisfaction with life, those who reported higher belief in witchcraft also reported lower satisfaction with life than those who reported lesser belief in witchcraft. This finding could be attributed to the span of control on one's life. Those who belief in witchcraft feels they have less control over their life and their health (in most cultures over their wealth) than those who believed otherwise.

Evaluative Wellbeing Lower for Sub-Saharan Africans Who Believe in Witchcraft

On which step of the ladder would you say you personally feel you stand at this time, assuming that the higher the step the better you feel about your life, and the lower the step the worse you feel about it? Which step comes closest to the way you feel?

	Average life evaluation rating among believers	Average life evaluation rating among those who don't believe
No formal education	3.8	4.3
One to eight years of education	4.2	4.5
Nine or more years of education	4.6	5.1
Living comfortably on present income	5.0	5.5
Getting by	4.8	5.3
Finding it difficult	4.2	4.6
Finding it very difficult on present income	3.8	4.3
Ages 15 to 18	4.3	5.0
Ages 19 to 29	4.4	4.8
Ages 30 to 45	4.3	4.7
Ages 46 and older	4.1	4.7
Poorest 20%	3.7	4.0

Surveys conducted between April and December 2009

GALLUP

As stated earlier, in witchery cultural belief, disease and illness are attributed to punishment from the gods or supernatural being rather than naturalistic causations; resulting in a greater sense of victimization by the gods for those who believe in witchcraft than those who believe otherwise. Study shows that witchery culture is a way of life for many people, especially in developing countries. There were several examples of negative and deadly implications of belief in witchcraft on public health and properties. Horrific killings, rape and humiliation in the name of witchery culture have also been reported around the world in the recent years.

As much as I tried to avoid making this discussion about the practice of and belief in witchcraft, I found it almost impossible to talk about the impact of cultural belief on public health without mentioning some senseless killings and harms imposed on our citizens as a result of belief in witchcraft. In July 5, 2013, the Kenyan police reported that at least 20 elderly people were killed each month in the little village of Kilifi Local government area after being accused of witchcraft by their kinsmen. Earlier in June 2009, 5 elderly people were burnt alive in front of the villagers in Kisii, Kenya.

In a village in Zambia in March 2013, two elderly people were axed to death by their relative who believed the elderly men were witches (a 63 year old woman and an 89 year old man). In another village in Zimbabwe, two elderly women died after being forced to drink a poisonous "portion" by their kinsmen who accused them of witchcraft.

In April 2003, a man was beheaded in a village in Uganda after being accused of witchcraft by his family members. In one region of Congo in DR Congo, 800 people were reported killed by their kinsmen after being accused of witchcraft. According to Amnesty International, between 1994 through 1998 more than 5,000 people were killed in Tanzania in a 4 year long witch hunt. 80% of the victims were elderly women killed by young men ages 16 – 35 years old.

This pattern of senseless killing continues in different parts of Africa. The Red Cross organization reported that more than 50 Albinos were murdered for their body parts in East Africa in 2009. According to the report, Albino's body parts, especially the fingers and genitals, are in high demand on the black market. In some part of Africa, they believe that Albino body parts contain magical powers and are used in witchcraft.

In all these killings, the questions we failed to ask are: What were the victims being accused of? What is the villager's procedure for confirming allegation of witchcraft before imposing death sentence on those victims? What makes them believe that their victims were witches and responsible for what they were being accused?

Having spent more than 25 years of my life in Africa, here is what I know; when people mismanage their business fund, they blame it on witchcraft. When someone, especially, rich person dies in a village, they blame it on the poor man or woman living in that community as being responsible for the rich person's death (witch). If someone dies in an auto accident in the city, the kinsmen accuse the elderly poor man or woman in the village of witchcraft and being responsible for the mishap.

In fact, the problem of misrepresentation of disease etiology is not only practiced in African countries. In many parts of Asia, disease epidemics and other Mother Nature events such as Tsunami, flooding, tornado have also been credited to witchcraft. Unrelated events such as failure in examination, loss of election, loss of job, unemployment and difficulty finding work, especially after graduation from a high institution, has been cited as an act of witchcraft. In many parts of Africa, when a married woman fails to conceive a child within months after marriage, or in most cases suffers a miscarriage or lose the baby before full term (still birth), witchcraft is cited for such misfortunes. Rather than seeking medical remedy to the problem, the couple tends to rely on rituals and consultations of witch doctors to counter the influence of the enemy witchcraft.

Unfortunately, the fruitless pain, financial loss, humiliation and emotional stress the couples (especially the women) are subjected to by the witch doctors cause more harm to their reproductive system, marital relationship, family etc., than childlessness. Sometimes it actually leads to break ups, accusations, and even death of innocent people. It is possible, that the actual problem is a hormone imbalance.

As the founder of Youth Arise Global Outreach Mission, I have travelled to different parts of the world in the past few years empowering and motivating the youths all over the world. One of the countries I have visited more often is the West African country of Sierra Leone. A decade-long Sierra Leonean civil war (1991 -2002) brought about a long lasting psychological devastation on the people of Serra Leone, more than a decade after the war ended.

Public health speaking, the end of civil war marks the beginning, if not the continuation of the psychological impact of war. Reports of surveys conducted on women in 2011 (almost a decade later) by Physicians for Human Rights depicts that 94% of the women rated their mental health as "poor or fair" while 28 % report experiencing suicidal thoughts or feelings. According to World Health Organization, over 100,000 Sierra Leoneans over 12 years of age were severely depressed, about 50,000 people living in Sierra Leone had demonstrated some kind of psychological disorder while more than 200,000 people reported some form of substance abuse.

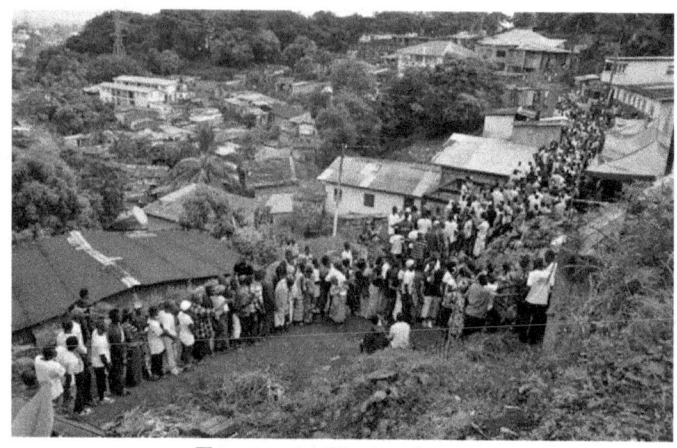

Freetown, Sierra Leone.

The statistics above is not surprisingly abnormal for a post-war country. It is a classic example of Post-Traumatic Stress Disorder (PSTD). What is of utmost concern is the lack of readiness of the leaders of Sierra Leone to address the issue of public health now and in years to come. With the level of chronic shortage of medical personnel (nurses and physicians) in the country, especially in the field of Psychiatry, more needs to be done by the public health professionals in creating awareness and mass education in the area of psychological health and wellbeing, depressive symptoms and mental health disorder.

Majority of the Serra Leoneans believe that mental health is somehow an imposed punitive on humans by a supernatural being (God); the resultant effect of such belief is ignorant unwillingness to seek medical help. Most people in the city of Freetown believe that mental health is a nemesis resulting from someone's past evil act. Due to the people's belief that mental illness is an act of payback or punitive from God, the people rather turn to the witch doctors for medical or healing help thereby unintentionally delaying or escalating the condition. Lack of public health education on mental health disorders, prevention and possible treatments has resulted in waste and loss of precious lives; some people are sincerely seeking for help but unfortunately in wrong places.

It is obvious that there is a chronic shortage of medical infrastructure and know-how in most developing countries; however, doing nothing is not the prescription for this illness. Public health education will enhance our knowledge of some of these diseases and reduce victim stigmatization. This information will equip the reader with the knowledge necessary to disarm witchery cultural belief in terms of disease etiology, prevention and control, rather than "glorifying" the witches for diseases and illness. It will also help you to identify symptoms of silent killer diseases, and "kill it before it kills you."

CHAPTER 3
THE SILENT KILLER

"There is a time for everything; a time to be born and a time to die.... (Ecclesiastes 3:1-2)

To some of us who have lost a loved one or know someone who has, you may wish the "time" was written on a stone, visible and readable for everyone who cares to know. With due credit given to the evolution of medical sciences, we can now "predict" a time to be born when the conception has already taken place, and to some degree a time to die when the patient is already ill with some kind of terminal disease/illness. Knowing the time to be born enables the family to prepare for the arrival of the new "Angel." In fact, knowing the sex of the baby makes it even easier for the family to buy the right color of clothing and bedding. Knowing the time to die reduces the emotional distortion, confusion and degree of pain on the bereaved as they prepare their "home" early enough.

For family with loved ones living outside of the states and country, they can all come home and see their loved one before his or her last breath. For the sick loved one, he or she will have the opportunity to address his family, make any final adjustments to his will, pray for his family, bless them and kiss them goodbye. That sounds like a perfect life! Sometimes I wish it is always like that, some of us who did not have the opportunity to hug, kiss, and squeeze our parents or spouse before their departure would seize one more opportunity to do so.

Unfortunately, we live in a time when the person you were with yesterday failed to return your phone call the next day, not because they didn't want to, but because they died. We live in a time when a driver at a traffic light or in a traffic jam cannot move when the traffic moves because he/she died while in the traffic jam. We live in a time when a man walking to his car at the parking lot, falls down beside his car and dies. We live in a time when a man wakes up in the morning with pain in his right eye; and by evening the other eye is watery, pink and painful. Couple of days later his vision turns from blurred to blind. They are here; the silent killer diseases!

In a village in Eastern Nigeria, a man bought a new car in the city where he resides; drove from Lagos to his village (10 – 12 hours' drive) to celebrate the new car with his kinsmen. They had an all-night party and few days later he was on his way back to Lagos. His trip back was safe and successful but 3 days later he was found dead in his apartment in Lagos - no injury, no robbery and no gun wound. The whole village was literally on fire with different conspiracy theories concerning his death. Similarly, in other part of Africa, the youth took to the street and at the end of the day; a couple in his village were accused of witchcraft and was murdered by an angry mob. The joy of the new car immediately turned sour; like a chemical chain reaction, hatred begat hatred and killing begat more killing.

Unfortunately, there are silent killers among us. As frightening as it may sound, the silent killers are neither human nor witchcraft. They are diseases! Medically speaking, it is obvious that the man in the story died of a heart attack aggravated by stress from more than 20 hours of driving.

Silent killers, for lack of a better definition, are described as those medical conditions that produce minimum or no symptoms but are capable of causing death if not recognized and treated immediately.

Despite technological advancement in the field of medical sciences in some developed countries, silent killer diseases still rate as the number one killer of both men and women in the developed countries. In Africa and other developing countries, while we are still awaiting a healthcare "Messiah", silent killer diseases lives and sleeps in our bedrooms, and eat their supper unnoticed.

Traditional and cultural beliefs, especially those that attribute disease to witchcraft, tends to make some developing countries a hideout for silent killer diseases. Due to belief and attributing disease epidemics to witchcraft, people rather consult witch doctors for the unexplained death of their loved ones. As a result, silent killer diseases go unnoticed, blameless and unpunished for their crime. A majority of diseases related to lifestyle are mostly diagnosed at an advanced stage, therefore, are referred to as silent killers. The silent killer diseases tend to disguise their warning signs and in most cases they either have symptoms similar to those of other less fatal diseases or even subtle symptoms difficult to detect but capable of causing death. Around the globe, silent killer diseases strike more than 10 million people each year and there are more than 100,000 deaths as a result of these diseases.

Our environment plays a very important role in our living. What we eat and breathe has a direct impact on our health. In some parts of the developing countries, environmental pollution is a way of life for many. In villages with no pipe water, people bathe and swim inside the same stream serving as a source of drinking water for the whole community. Are you still wondering why Onchocerciasis (River blindness) was a major public health problem in some parts of the continent? A friend of mine visited his uncle in one of the villages some years ago and the uncle's wife cooked him some special traditional meal. Later that night, he came down with vomiting and diarrhea. A few days later, the whole family was summoned by the traditional rulers and elders of the village because he accused his brother's wife of poisoning him. The truth is, he suffered from food poisoning but it was probably not intentional poisoning by his uncle's wife. It is possible that the vegetable or one of the ingredients used in cooking the food was contaminated, which could be in part as a result of the environmental conditions. It is not witchcraft; it is the silent killer disease.

Heart disease, hypertension, different eye diseases, tetanus, tuberculosis and diabetes are among major silent killer diseases that are discussed in this book. World Health Organization in 2012 reported that heart disease was the number one silent killer disease; with main risk factors such hypertension, smoking, and high cholesterol. More than 249 million people around the globe suffer from diabetes each year and about 3.2 million of them die due to diabetes related complications. We need to be enlightened and refocus our efforts on the war against silent killer diseases, rather than witchcraft.

We need to identify the signs, symptoms, risk factors, causes and possible prevention of some "Silent killer" diseases and understand the common known treatment options for these diseases.

In most developing countries, due to financial restraints and the belief that illness is as a result of a witch curse, people only consult medically trained physicians when they are literally "half dead." In Nigeria, Cameroon and Sierra Leone for example,

34

there are currently no functioning medical health insurance systems that serve regular citizens. Self-medication is the first line of medical care in time of illness for most people living in these countries. The ease of access to medication (prescription and non-prescription drugs) could be seen as both good and bad depending on the situation. Unfortunately, a majority of drug dispensers in most of these countries (commonly called Chemist or even doctors) are not trained medical professionals. Some of them are just locally trained skilled drug dispensers with no college degree.

In order to save money or manage the little funds available, most people go to a standalone laboratory for testing and then bring the laboratory result to the dispensers for prescription. In some cases, depending on the city or location, these "local drug dispensers" diagnose and dispense medication for the patients without proper laboratory examination. There is actually no culprit in this situation. Most families in developing countries have to decide what is of high priority when the choice is to either pay for food or pay for medical care.

On a good note, it is important to add that some of these drug dispensers have spent lots of years in the business and have actually gained lots of experience. Over the years, however, they were the only alternative for persons needing medical care. Despite their lack of medical qualification and training, they have provided leverage for the poor people struggling to decide whether to pay for food or take their love ones to the hospital.

Since the dispensers depend largely on common symptoms to diagnose their patients, providing them with knowledge of symptoms, causes and treatment of some of the silent killer diseases will be an added advantage to their diagnostic skills; and help save lives by empowering both the people and the drug dispensers.

CHAPTER 4
SILENT KILLER #1 : DIABETES MELLITUS

The name diabetes mellitus commonly referred to as diabetes originated from Greek and Latin words; *diabetes* means siphon or passing through something and *mellitus* (Latin) means honeyed or sweet. In fact, in most African languages, the disease Diabetes is commonly translated as sweet or sugar-related diseases or wealthy people diseases. This is because some believe that you have to be wealthy to eat sugary or sweetened food stuff that is capable of resulting in the disease diabetes. Unfortunately, medical science have proven that concept wrong.

Meanwhile, Diabetes mellitus is a condition that disrupts the proper utilization of blood (glucose) sugar. Blood sugar (Glucose) plays a vital role in your body's metabolism and general health as it is a major source of energy for the body's cells that operates and controls the activities that goes on in your body.

When your body fails in its responsibility to control the amount of sugar produced and distributed in your body; it results in a condition (illness) called diabetes. When your body allows excess glucose into your system due to the disease diabetes, it can lead to either death (if not controlled) or result in other sister diseases. There are different types of diabetes: Type 1 and Type 2 depending on the degree of elevation of blood sugar in your system.

SYMPTOMS OF DIABETES

The degree of elevation of your blood sugar (glucose) from normal determines the type of diabetes diagnosed. Some of the known symptoms of diabetes are as follows:

- Unexplained frequent urination
- Fatigue
- Blurred vision
- Excessive hunger
- Ease of infection or frequent infection such as skin or bladder infections.
- Low-healing sores are also attributed to diabetes
- Elevated ketones during basic urinalyses shows that a breakdown of muscle and fat is taking place in the body. This is usually as a result of little or not enough insulin in the body.

It is important to note that in most cases, depending on the individual, some of the symptoms of diabetes may not manifest in its early stages resulting in a condition called Type 2 diabetes. The good news is that the type 2 diabetes, which also happens to be the most common, is preventable. However symptoms of type 1 diabetes are usually quick and severe.

If you notice any of these symptoms, it is highly recommended that you see your physician for checkup.

CAUSES OF DIABETES

Diabetes occurs as a result of glucose imbalance in the body. In a normal healthy (diabetes free) body, the pancreas gland secretes a hormone called insulin into the body (bloodstream), and as the insulin circulates through the bloodstream it deposits and control the amount of sugar circulating through the body cells. There are different factors that could contribute to blood sugar abnormalities- for example, eating too much, being sick or not taking enough glucose-lowering medication.

An imbalance in the amount of insulin deposited in the body by the pancreas gland affects the amount of sugar deposited into the bloodstream at a particular point in time. The body stores its sugar in the liver; therefore, whenever the level of insulin in the bloodstream is low, the liver reprocesses the stored sugar (glycogen) into glucose. This is what happens especially when you starve your body of food for some time.

In some abnormal cases, your body's immune system which is supposed to fight harmful bacteria that enters your body from your environment, turns and destroys the cell that produces insulin in your body. At this time, your body's ability to transport sugar through the bloodstream (by insulin) is destroyed leaving your body with sugar build up in the bloodstream. This condition leads to, Type 1-diabetes. There are different factors that could contribute to the occurrence of this abnormal event; witchcraft is not one of them.

In most cases, the body cell tends to resist the action (movement) of insulin around the body and the pancreas gland is unable to produce enough insulin to overcome this resistance. During pregnancy for example, the body's resistance to insulin gets worst due to actions of the hormone produced by the placenta, resulting in a lack of sugar in vital areas of your body where sugar is needed. This condition leads to Type 2-diabetes.

Factors that could contribute to type 1 and 2-diabetes includes; genetic makeup (if your parents or siblings have diabetes, your chance of having diabetes increases), presence of damaged immune system due to viral disease or chemical substances. The consumption of certain food substances especially those low in vitamin D is also attributed to risk factors of diabetes.

In fact, studies by MAYO clinics claimed that *early consumption of cow's milk or exposure to cereals before 4 months of age* could increase the risk of diabetes. Body weight and inactivity (lack of exercise) is another known risk factor for diabetes. The fatty tissue in your body restricts the normal circulation of insulin in your bloodstream. Physical activity helps your body literally "work out" glucose resulting in body cell sensitivity to insulin.

Exercise is highly recommended-at minimum three times per week. While, growing up in Nigeria in the 90's, a majority of Nigerians did not have pipe water and we had to travel between 8-10 kilometers to fetch 5-10 gallons of stream water. It was not a good experience, but that was good exercise.

Finally, your age, history of certain diseases and racial background is a risk factor for certain types of diabetes. Study shows that blacks are at a higher risk of type 2-diabetes and the risk of diabetes increase as we grow older.

If your blood pressure is higher than 140/90mm Hg, you are at high risk of type 2-diabetes. Also, low level of good cholesterol (High-density lipoprotein) HDL level 35mg/dL is a high risk factor for type 2-diabetes.

COMPLICATIONS OF DIABETES

In general, complications associated with diabetes and other killer diseases increase as the disease lingers in your body undiagnosed and untreated. In most cases, the conspiracy theory that witchcraft is the cause of this illness creates an avenue for increased complication especially when the patient consults witchdoctors (Vodoo master) for help rather than medical experts. Complications from abnormality of blood sugar (diabetes) gradually become life-threatening as it affects other body organs. Undiagnosed and untreated diabetes increases the risk of heart diseases such as coronary artery with chest pain, heart attack and stroke.

Because most diabetes diseases result from sugar imbalance in the body, excess sugar in any part of the body could result in damage to body nerve especially in the leg (toes) resulting in numbness, ulcer and blisters, tingling and burning or pain.

Depending on the length of time the diabetes disease is left untreated, it could lead to total loss of the feeling of sensation in the affected toes, even erectile dysfunction due to nerve damage. Diabetes disease could also affect the kidney by destroying the glomeruli (tiny blood vessel that filter waste from the blood) and probably complete kidney failure. Diabetes also affects the part of the eyes called Retina by damaging the blood vessel that supplies body nutrients to the eye. Retina is the spot in the eyes where images are formed. Damage to the retina could result to partial or total blindness. Other eye diseases such as glaucoma and cataract are worsened by diabetes. Lack of knowledge of symptoms and possible complications from this disease establish the conspiracy theory citing witchcraft as the possible cause. To every abnormal event or situation, a possible cause must be attributed.

Unfortunately, when it comes to public health and disease prevention, lack of knowledge does more harm than good as it results in out of control epidemics and disease spread. The World Health Organization reported this morning that the lack of knowledge and risk factors for Ebola disease has made it very difficult to try to contain the spread of this killer disease. The problem in the case of illnesses such as diabetes and its complications is that the longer the false causative theory leading to wrong treatment options lingers, the more life threatening the complications from the disease.

Finally diabetes during pregnancy (gestational diabetes) could be dangerous, affecting the mother or the baby and sometimes both. In most cases, women with gestational diabetes actually deliver healthy babies. Meanwhile, diabetes condition and its complications during pregnancy could become life threatening if the disease is untreated. One of the complications of gestational diabetes is that your baby tends to grow larger than normal (macrosomia) due to excess glucose across the baby's placenta. In this case, delivery through normal birth could be either very difficult or impossible resulting in Caesura-section (C-section). In gestational diabetes, your best option is to work with your physician to ensure the condition is managed even after delivery, as untreated gestational diabetes could result in a baby's death before or shortly after delivery.

DIAGNOSIS OF DIABETES

Since diabetes is a blood sugar disease. Diagnosis of diabetes occurs through monitoring of blood sugar. As earlier stated, some of the known symptoms of diabetes do not appear early enough, while some appears suddenly. Checking the blood sugar regularly will help detect abnormalities in blood sugar level. The American Diabetes Association has recommended that anyone with a body mass index higher than 25 regardless of their age or race, who also has additional risk factors stated earlier in this book such as high blood pressure, history of diabetes in the family, delivered baby higher than 4.0 kilogram or 9 pounds should be tested regularly. Also, anyone older than 45 years old should be tested, and if the initial result shows normal or no elevated blood sugar, the individual should be tested every three years for blood sugar.

A blood glucose test could be done either randomly or while fasting. For random sugar level test, if your blood sugar level during blood test shows 200 milligram per deciliter (mg/dL) or 11.1 millimoles per liter (mmol/L) or higher, that suggests diabetes. It is recommended that you consult your physician immediately. For fasting sugar level test, if your blood sugar level test shows between 100 and 125 mg/dL (5.6 and 6.9 mmol/L) that is considered pre-diabetes. However, if your blood sugar test shows 126 mg/dL (7 mmol/L) you will be diagnosed with diabetes and you must consult your physician. Most physicians will send you for a retest in order to confirm your laboratory result before starting treatment.

For pregnant women, your physician normally tests you for gestational diabetes early in your pregnancy. However, this gets scarier and scarier knowing that in most developing countries, pregnant women receive little or no prenatal care. In most cases, some women wait until their third trimester before consulting their physician, while some just show up in the maternity ward when they are already in labor, not because they despise medical care, but because of the lack of financial capabilities to seek and pay for medical care. In this situation, the culprit silent killer disease goes unnoticed, undiscovered and un-convicted.

PREVENTION, CONTROL AND TREATMENT OF DIABETES

Treatment and control of all types of diabetes is achieved mostly through blood sugar monitoring, insulin or other oral medication. However, maintaining a healthy lifestyle such as weight watching, and eating a healthy diet is key to the successful treatment and control of all types of diabetes. You should avoid saturated and trans-fats, sweets and sugary foods. Eat varieties of fruits, vegetables, low-fat dairy products, beans and whole grain foods each day.

In most parts of developing countries, alcohol consumption is a likely hobby to many unemployed farmers and idle persons. Alcohol (especially the locally brewed), due to the high level of ethanol and impurities, is especially toxic to diabetic patients and can worsen diabetic nerve damage, decrease vision and high blood pressure.

Studies reported by Mayo clinic suggests that our diets should be centered on more fruits, vegetables and whole grains — foods that are high in nutrition and fiber and low in fat and calories — and cut down on animal products, refined carbohydrates and sweets.

The problem with eating healthy, especially for those living in the developing countries, are that a majority of the people have little or no choice of what to eat and what not to eat. While most of us living in developed countries are conscious of our diet; whether it is balanced or not, a majority of people living in the poverty trodden areas of the developing countries have just a little to fill their stomach. Poverty and lack of enough to eat makes it difficult to control diabetes among such a vulnerable population. Do not wait until you are diagnosed with diabetes before you start watching your diet. Remember the adage…"prevention is better than cure…"

Among other preventive measures for diabetes, exercise has been proven to be very effective in managing and preventing diabetes. Physical activities that constitute exercise is energy demanding, and helps to lower blood sugar by transporting sugar to the body cells where it is converted and used for energy. If you have certain cardiac conditions or illness, it is recommended that you consult your doctor on the kind and type of exercise regimen you should embark on. There are other medical or treatment options available in developed countries for treatment of diabetes which are beyond the scope of this book.

At this point, you should be able to differentiate between Type 1 and Type 2-diabetes and their risk factors. In general, prevention of diabetes has both good and bad news. The bad news is that Type 1-diabetes cannot be prevented while the Type 2-diabetes and the gestational diabetes can be prevented. The good news is that the same healthy lifestyle choices that help to treat type 2 and other types of diabetes, could also help reduce the prevalence of type 1-diabetes.

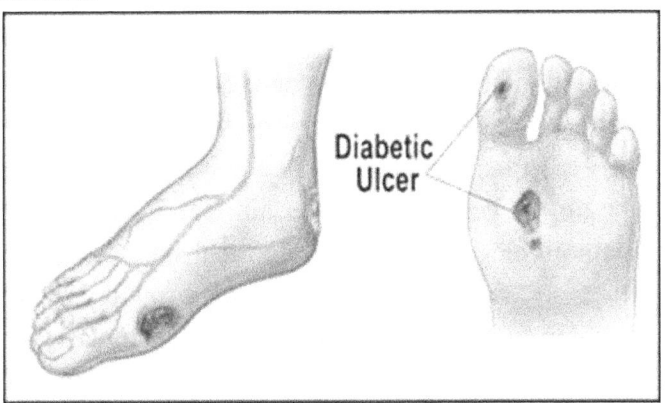

Poorly controlled diabetes also places you at serious increased risk of heart attack and stroke as well as blindness and amputation

NATURAL REMEDIES FOR TREATMENT OF DIABETICS

Where possible, seek out natural remedies for prevention or treatment of some silent killer diseases. For example, the plant foods below are sometimes used for treatment of type 2 diabetes treatment.

- Brewer's yeast
- Buckwheat
- Broccoli and other related greens
- Cinnamon
- Cloves
- Coffee
- Okra
- Peas
- Fenugreek seeds
- Sage

Nutritionists claim that most of the plant food listed above are rich in fiber, vitamins, and minerals, which are important and good for people living with diabetes. Studies show that certain plant foods such as cinnamon, cloves, and coffee can enhance the body's ability to fight inflammation and help insulin. Cinnamon extracts can increase sugar metabolism, trigger insulin release, thereby affecting metabolism of cholesterol. Clove oil extracts (eugenol) have been found to improve the function of insulin and to lower glucose, cholesterol, LDL, and triglycerides. This oil is also used in the treatment of/dental care (toothache).

CHAPTER 5
SILENT KILLER #2: HEART DISEASE AND STROKE

The term "heart attack" refers to any incident or event that causes a permanent injury or damage to the heart muscles or tissues. Another name for heart attack is myocardial infarction which is interpreted as "death of heart muscle". "Myo" means muscle and "cardial" means heart. Although there are several scientific attributions to heart attack, most common heart attacks occur when there is abnormality of flow of blood into the heart region through the artery called coronary, as a result, causing damage to the heart muscle.

This disease made our list of silent killers due to its fatal nature. However, the scariest part of this disease is that it can occur at any point in time with little or no symptoms. That is why in most parts of Africa and other developing countries, people tend to attribute heart attacks to witchcraft.

SYMPTOMS OF HEART ATTACK

Like any other silent killer disease, the ability to identify symptoms associated with heart attack, can help the patient make a life-saving decision. There is a saying in Africa that what you don't know will not hurt you. I think silent killer diseases have proven that to be wrong. What you don't know can also kill you.

Common symptoms associated with heart attack are:

- Feeling of anxiety
- Trouble sleeping
- Shortness of breath
- Sweating or cold sweat
- Lightheadedness
- Tightness (especially around the chest area)
- Squeezing sensation in the chest or even the arm. In most cases, the squeezing sensation spreads from one point to other areas.

It is important to note that symptoms of heart attack may vary from one individual to another and you may not experience all the symptoms listed above at one time. Another scary point about heart attacks is that the severity of the symptom varies; while some people do not notice any symptom at all, for some, the first symptom they notice results in an actual heart attack. Heart attacks can occur at any place or time; whether you are at work or on vacation. You probably knew someone or know someone who knew someone that died literally on a steering wheel while driving. Someone stopped on a red light or in a traffic "jam" known as "go slow" in some parts of Africa, while waiting for traffic flow to resume, died right on the steering wheel.

The severity and suddenness of a heart attack is what leads to the common practice of attributing the devastation of this disease to witchcraft in some parts of the developing countries. The danger here is that when we attribute the damage caused by silent killer diseases to witchcraft, medically recommended precautions (such as voluntary testing) will not be taken to prevent future occurrences or potential danger to other relatives. Although heart attack is a silent killer disease, some people are fortunate enough to experience the symptoms for days, weeks or even months. However, if the warning signs of heart attack are neglected, sudden death is inevitable.

The most common and earliest symptom of heart attack is chest pain know as (Angina). It is commonly caused by exertion resulting in temporary decrease in blood flow to the heart; another reason having good rest often is a recommended practice that can save lives. It is important to note also, that there is a difference between heart attack and cardiac arrest.

Cardiac arrest occurs when an electrical disturbance in your heart causes the pumping action of the heart to cease resulting in temporary shortage of blood supply to the body. The science of heart attack and that of cardiac arrest is beyond the scope of this book, but it might benefit the reader to know that heart attack can result in cardiac arrest.

RESPONDING TO HEART ATTACK

There is nothing more frustrating than being a witness to a heart attack episode but have no idea what to do to try to save the person. The first and basic first response to heart attack is to begin Cardiopulmonary Resuscitation (CPR) procedure. The bad news is that it is highly recommended that you be trained to do CPR. The good news is that you can still do CPR even if you have not been officially trained. The training takes less than 2 hours and you can receive the training in every local hospital, health center, fire station etc. CPR will help resume the flow of oxygen to the body and brain.

For the benefit of your commitment to reading this book, here is your quick overview of how to perform CPR:

- You should begin CPR with chest compressions. Press down about 2 inches (5 centimeters) on the person's chest for each compression at a rate of about 100 a minute. If you've been trained in CPR, check the person's airway and deliver rescue breaths after every 30 compressions. If you haven't been trained, continue doing only compressions until help arrives.

- You can actually save a life with that quick overview…..

Trained professionals can use an automated external defibrillator (AED), which shocks the heart back into a normal rhythm to provide emergency treatment before a person having a heart attack reaches the hospital. However, in the absence of an AED, please continue chest compression. If there is someone else in the room or the area, send that person to go look for help or call 911 (emergency responders) if it is available. In some countries and some areas like where I grew up, that number does not exist.

CAUSES OF HEART ATTACK

The body's arteries are like electrical cables that transmit electricity to and from power stations to your home. The difference here is that the arteries, unlike the electric cables, have a hollow passage where fluid such as blood passes. Depending on what is being transported through the arteries, there are usually deposits from the substance left on the walls of the artery. Unfortunately the artery becomes narrowed, over a period of time, from the buildup of various substances that are being transported by the fluid flowing through the artery. One of the common and dangerous substances that are being deposited on the walls of the artery is the cholesterol. The buildup of cholesterol and other substances on the artery wall results in a condition called atherosclerosis. In a lay man term, the hollow space in the artery that allows for passage of blood pumped from the heart becomes so narrow that it is difficult for blood to pass through- (imagine heavy traffic in the streets of Mombasa,

Kenya or Lagos, Nigeria). It is absolutely difficult for vehicles even emergency vehicles to pass through.

Heart attack can also occur as a result of spasm of the coronary artery resulting in a partial or total shut down of blood flow to parts of the heart muscles. Coronary artery spasm refers to the "tightening" of muscles around the artery in the heart region; causing the narrowing of the artery and thereby inhibiting blood flow through the artery. Coronary artery spasm is not a lengthy episode; they are brief and temporary, however it could lead to other complications. This disease made the list of our silent killers because the symptoms of coronary artery (mostly chest pain, pain on the left side of the chest, feeling of constriction, chest tightness) spasms go unnoticed, but could lead to heart attack.

The most common cause of coronary spasm could be attributed to high cholesterol and hypertension. Common risk factors associated with coronary artery spasm include smoking, use of illegal drug like cocaine, extreme stress and extreme cold.

RISK FACTORS FOR HEART ATTACK

As we identify the symptoms associated with silent killer diseases, another thing we try to do is to provide you with the information that will enable you to make educated decisions (in terms of their lifestyle) that will help prevent the chance of occurrence of these diseases.

Everything we have discussed so far about the silent killer disease, heart attack, has to do with malfunction of the artery. That means, in order to prevent heart diseases, we should literally invest in activities/lifestyle that will help us care for our heart's arteries.

Common risk factors for heart attack include unwanted buildup of fatty deposits in the arteries all over the body. Reducing the chance of fatty deposit in your body will reduce the chance of heart attack.

Age

Between the age of 45 and 55 years old the risk of heart attack increases both for men and women respectively. Unfortunately, your geographical location does not exempt you from the risk of fatty buildup. For most people in the developing countries all they care about is any food that will help quench the torture of hunger and bring their "tummy" peace while most people in the developed country have high accessibility to easily affordable "fast food" that is increasing the risk of fatty buildup in the arteries.

Tobacco Consumption

Direct or indirect (secondhand) smoking has damaging effects on the interior arteries walls. While some persons do not smoke per say, if they are constantly "hanging out" with friends and relatives who smoke (secondhand smoking) the effect is sure to be the same. The only difference is in the incubation period (time it will take before the effects manifest). Parents who smoke indoors in their home and cars successfully expose their children and relatives to secondhand smoke.

When the interior walls of the arteries is damaged through smoking, it becomes very easy for cholesterol and other poisonous substances to be deposited in the "crack" walls of the arteries and drastically reduce blood flow. Teenagers should be empowered to resist the peer pressure that has led to high rates of teenage smoking among our children.

High Blood Pressure

If diagnosed with high blood pressure, it is highly recommended that you work with your physician to ensure your blood pressure is constantly monitored. If uncontrolled, over time, the excessive pressure exerted in the arteries (high blood pressure) will damage the arteries that feed blood into the heart resulting to arteriosclerosis. This condition is worsened by other complications such as obesity, smoking, high cholesterol and even diabetes.

High Blood Cholesterol (Triglyceride)

The most significant and common deposit that narrows the hollow space of the artery is cholesterol. Unfortunately, a majority of the food we eat all contain some kind of cholesterol. According to the American Heart Association, there are two classes of cholesterol - the "bad" cholesterol known as Low-density lipoprotein (LDL) and the "good" cholesterol known as High-density lipoprotein (HDL). While high levels of the "bad" cholesterol in your body poses the risk of heart attack, high levels of the "good" cholesterol (HDL) in your body protects you from heart attack.

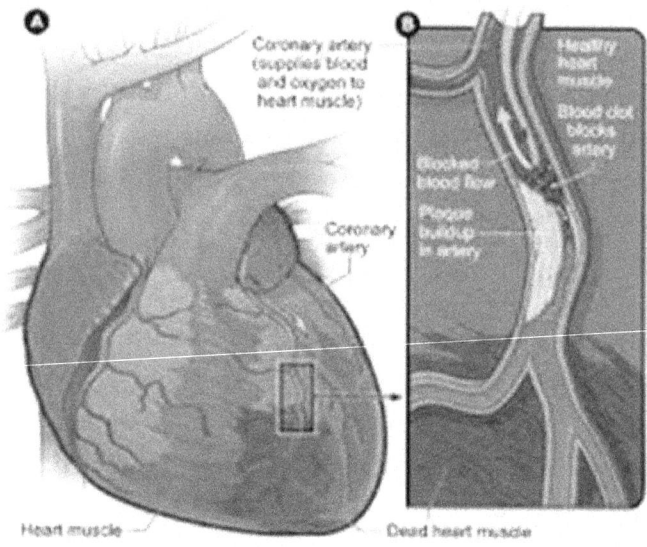

Other risk factors for heart attack includes: diabetes (as discussed earlier) and family history of heart attack. If your parents or siblings suffered from heart attack, your chances of heart attack are higher than your other friends with no family history of heart attack. That is why it is important that you understand your family medical history and adhere to lifestyle that has the potential to reduce the risk. Unfortunately, for most people in the developing country who have no record of diagnosis or prognosis of family members, the silent killers could operate silently for a very long time causing diseases or complications that could potentially lead to death due to lack of knowledge.

In all of this, the signs of ignoramus are being blamed on witchcraft making prevention almost impossible. When people site witchcraft as the probable cause of death of their loved ones due to lack of knowledge of probable symptoms of silent killer diseases, family members who are still alive do not get checked out because of the conspiracy theory. This ignoramus negligence could potentially result in the escalation of the effect of silent killer diseases, since no preventive measure is in place.

AFTER A HEART ATTACK

Heart attack is not without complication even if one survives the attack. The complications associated with heart attack actually occur during the episode itself. Some of the complications associated with heart attack include:

ARRHYTHMIAS

This refers to the abnormal heart rhythms which are as a result of possible damage caused to the heart muscle from the heart attack. In some cases, arrhythmias could even lead to death.

HEART FAILURE

The heart tends to "fail" during a heart attack since the amount of damaged caused to the tissues in the heart in most cases could be so severe that the heart muscle is unable to pump blood out of the heart to other parts of the body. Heart failure could be a temporary problem; in some cases, and once the heart recovers from the attack the condition normalizes. In most cases, the condition fails to recover resulting in a chronic and permanent damage to the heart.

Other complications of heart attack involve: rupture of the muscular walls or heart muscle, heart valves damage, etc.

PREVENTION AND CONTROL OF HEART ATTACK

Your lifestyle plays an important role when it comes to the health of your heart. To maintain a healthy and strong heart will require you to embark on a lifestyle that reduces the introduction of unwanted substances, including stress, into the arteries. The following measures will help prevent or aid your recovery from a heart attack.

Say No to Smoking

Smoking cessation could be challenging, but quitting could increase your overall quality of life. Smoking cessation is not a lone ranger war. You need support of other people especially your doctor, friends and family. Above all, stay away from any source of second hand smoke.

Prevention, Prevention and Prevention

There is a popular saying in Africa that "prevention is better than cure." Public health wise, this statement is absolutely true. However, due to the deteriorating public health system in some developing countries, people do not consult their physician until they are literally at the point of death, not because they want to die, but because they lack funding for medical checkup or treatment.

Otherwise, checking your blood pressure and cholesterol level regularly will help prevent the risk of heart attack. You doctor should be able to prescribe changes to your diet or medication if at any point during a regular checkup your blood pressure and cholesterol is high.

Exercise, Exercise and Exercise

Exercising regularly will enhance your muscles especially those around your heart. As a result, your cardiologist (heart doctor) will recommend exercise as a rehabilitation program after heart attack, but most importantly as a preventive and control measure for another heart attack. Exercise helps maintain healthy weight, controls cholesterol and high blood pressure. When we hear exercise, some of us think of it in an Olympic perspective, not knowing that walking 30 minutes a day, 5 days a week can achieve tremendous result.

To maintain a healthy heart and control diabetes, you must also maintain healthy weight and eat healthy food. This combination is lacking for most persons. As stated earlier, too much fatty food is a dangerous recipe that can endanger the walls of the arteries to your heart.

Stress Management

Living in Africa or other developing countries imposes its own form of stress on its citizens. According to UNICEF, 22,000 children die each day due to poverty. And they "die quietly in some of the poorest villages on earth, far removed from the scrutiny and the conscience of the world. Being meek and weak in life makes these dying multitudes even more invisible in death." Of the 1.9 billion children from the developing world; 640 million are without adequate shelter (1 in 3); 400 million with no access to safe water (1 in 5); 270 million with no access to health services (1 in 7).

According to this report, South Asia and Sub-Saharan Africa shares the bulk of poverty in the world. Life itself in this part of the world is stressful, from weather and climatic conditions to the thought of what to eat and how to pay for the basic necessities of life. Managing ill-health and caring for sick loved ones drive the train of stress onto the freeway. It is important that we learn how to cope and manage stress because failure to do so opens the door for the "silent killer" to creep in. Most people turn to alcohol consumption as a means of coping with stress. That is too dangerous and could lead to invasion by silent killers and other uninvited guest into your heart's arteries.

TREATMENT OF HEART ATTACK

Following a heart attack episode, treatment should start right away. In places where there is Emergency Management Services (EMS) the treatments usually start inside the ambulance. Depending on the nature and severity of the heart attack, your doctor may prescribe drugs or recommend surgical procedure. Irrespective of the treatment method your doctor introduces, the aim is to gradually break up or totally prevent blood clots, inhibit ability of platelets and artery plaque, stabilize the plaque if already formed and prevent further damage to the heart muscle.

Whichever treatment option is selected by your doctor, the important factor here is timing. The treatment must be administered immediately and constant monitoring by the physician is necessary. I understand that a majority of you may live in cities with little or no access to physicians and emergency rooms, however, I believe this information will serve as a catalyst that will facilitate a discussion in the area of community health initiatives.

During a heart attack, your doctor is most likely to prescribe drugs such as Aspirin, Brilinta, and Plavix (that will help prevent blood clotting).

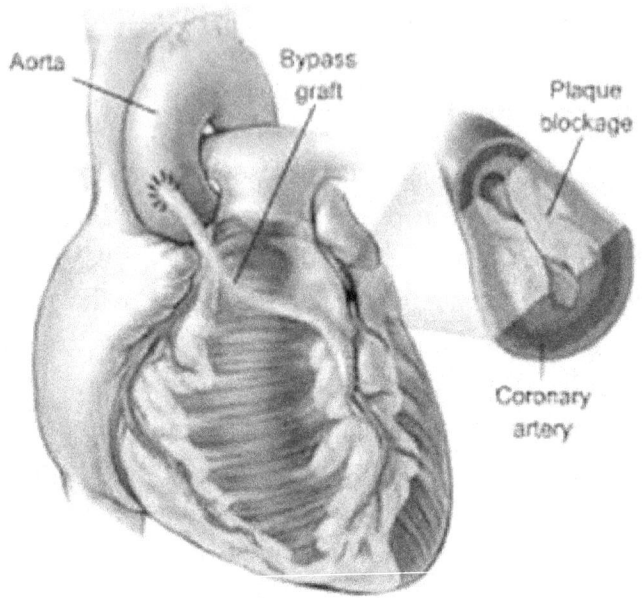

NATURAL REMEDY FOR TREATMENT AND CONTROL OF HEART DISEASE

Heart attacks, as we have learned so far, is one of the deadly silent killers and has the most potential to be diagnosed as witchcraft. Meanwhile, studies have shown that there are some common food items that have the ability to control or treat heart disease. Examples of recommended food items with remedial ingredients for heart disease are:

Bran Cereal

Bran cereal is known to be rich in fiber. Its nutritional value includes the ability to enhance and control cholesterol levels. Other food items such as beans (kidney and black bean), barley, oats, whole grains (brown rice and lentils) are high-fiber rich and can prevent heart disease by controlling cholesterol levels.

Olive Oil

Studies published by the American Heart Association and the American Dietetic Association recommend olive oil as a safe source of mono-unsaturated fat. The association highly recommends using olive oil for cooking rather than other forms of vegetable oil.

Peanut Butter

Peanut butter is known to be rich in Vitamin E. Study shows that 2 tablespoons of peanut butter could result in 1/3 of recommended daily intake of vitamin E. The problem here is that peanut butter (if eaten in excess, has the ability to result in weight gain). So if you are watching your weight, you need to watch the amount of peanut you consume.

Pecans

Pecan nuts nutritionally are known as an excellent source of Magnesium. It is highly recommended to maintain a healthy heart. Study shows that about 28 grams of pecan spread spinach salad can give you 1/3 of recommended daily allowance of this vital mineral.

Whole Wheat Bread

In 2012, after my regular annual checkup, my doctor recommended that I eat wheat bread instead of regular sweet white bread. At the beginning it sounded like punishment to me but as my taste buds got used to it, it is now difficult for me to eat regular bread. Wheat bread may not be as "yummy" if you just started eating it, but I highly recommend that you continue eating it due its known nutritional values.

In fact, spreading some grams of peanut butter on wheat bread gives you double portion of healthy heart food. Whole-wheat bread contains selenium, an antioxidant mineral that works with vitamin E to protect your heart.

Broccoli

Broccoli is a major source of Calcium and another heart-healthy nutrient. Milk as you already know is another calcium-rich food. The mineral calcium not only keeps your heart health, but also supports your bone health. Other sources of calcium found in your kitchen and around your garden are kale, salmon, figs, pinto beans and okra.

Salmon Fish

Salmon fish is known as a good source of Vitamin B12 and Omega-3 fatty acid. It is in fact highly recommended as part of your diet if you are at risk of heart disease. The irony of salmon and fishermen is that most of the fishermen who actually catch this fish in the water do not have the luxury to eat them. They rather sell them to the highest bidder and use the money to solve other needs at home that is likely unrelated to heart disease.

Orange and Strawberries

Vitamin C is an antioxidant vital to maintaining a happy heart. Oranges and strawberries are known major sources of vitamin C. ½ cup of sweet berry contains about 45 milligrams of the heart healthy vitamin C. Strawberries are also good source of fiber and potassium.

CHAPTER 6
SILENT KILLER #3: STROKES (CEREBRO-VASCULAR DISEASE)

At this point, you must have noticed that most of the diseases or conditions' affecting the heart is a result of restriction in blood flow causing variation in normal heart activities. Any form of abnormality in the functioning of the heart disrupts the entire circulatory system causing, in most cases, irreparable harm to the part of the body affected.

Cerebro-Vascular disease, popularly known as stroke, occurs when any of the conditions discussed earlier results in restricted or severely reduced blood flow in the brain region of the body; resulting in a shortage or complete absence of oxygen and other nutrients supplied through the blood to the brain. Unfortunately, unlike other parts of the body, the brain cells tend to start dying within minutes of lack of oxygen supply; making this condition (stroke) a medical emergency. Like other silent killer diseases, symptoms of stroke could go unnoticeable, however, early intervention in the event of a stroke could minimize the severity of its effect on the body. As terrifying as a stroke episode sounds, this condition can be prevented or treated; but of utmost importance is the knowledge of the symptoms of stroke.

SYMPTOMS OF STROKE

Your ability to identify signs and symptoms of some of these silent killer diseases is the difference between life and death. Some of the obvious symptoms of strokes are:

- Difficulty walking or exercising
- Dizziness
- Lack of balance or coordination
- Trouble with speaking and even to understand
- Sudden numbness, weakness or paralysis of some part of your body especially the face, arm or leg. Numbness or paralysis sometimes occurs in just one part of your body.
- Sudden blurred or blackened vision.
- Sudden severe headache

It is important to take note of the onset of these symptoms as your doctor may want to know how long you have had them to determine the best treatment for you. If the muscles in your arm cannot hold your arms up when you raise it, then, you need to see your doctor immediately. It is highly recommended to seek medical attention once you discover any of these symptoms. For those living in developed countries, you should dial 911 or any emergency number for medical attention.

In the event of a stroke, every minute that passes without medical treatment could result in the death of several body cells making it more difficult to resuscitate the victim. Unfortunately, in most developing countries hundreds of factors make prevention of a stroke difficult if not impossible during a stroke. Some of the factors making it difficult to save the victims include lack of access to good roads, proximity to the hospital, health centers, lack of functioning emergency medical services team (ambulance). Some of the health centers and clinics lack trained providers.

The most effective intervention during a stroke occurs within the first 3 hours of the symptoms. Every effort need to be made to ensure the victim sees a trained medical expert within the 3 hours window of the first stroke symptom.

CAUSES OF STROKE

As stated earlier, a stroke occurs when any of the conditions discussed earlier results in restricted or severely reduced blood flow into the brain region of the body; resulting in shortage or complete absence of oxygen and other nutrients supplied through the blood to the brain. In layman terms, lack of oxygen or essential nutrients starves the brain cells to death.

Stroke may occur as a result of blockage in the artery; a condition known as ischemic stroke (majority of stroke related visits to the doctor is as a result of ischemic stroke). There are two types of Ischemic stroke: Thrombotic stroke which occur due to blood clots formed in the artery as a result of fatty deposits in the artery resulting in restricted blood flow and Embolic stroke which occurs due to blood clots but the difference is that in this case, the blood clot occurs away from the brain.

A stroke can also occur as a result of a leak or bursting of a blood vessel (hemorrhagic stroke) referred to as "internal bleeding" in some local communities. There are two types of hemorrhagic strokes. Intracerebral hemorrhage occur when a blood vessel in the brain bursts and spills into the surrounding brain tissue that is not absorbed resulting in damage to the brain and Subarachnoid hemorrhage occurs when an artery on or near the surface of the brain bursts and spills into the space between the surface of the brain and the skull, resulting in erratic widening or narrowing of the blood vessel in the brain region.

Finally, strokes can result from temporary disruption of blood flow through the brain (transient ischemic attack). Some authors refer to transient ischemic attacks as a mini stroke since it is a brief episode of symptoms similar to those of stroke. Like other fully accredited transient stroke it is caused by temporary restriction in blood flow to parts of the brain.

RISK FACTORS FOR STROKE

A majority of diseases or conditions related to the artery or blood vessel dysfunction have common risk factors. The good news here is that as you strive to prevent one condition, you are actually preventing other conditions. The opposite is not so good as the condition that led to one could potentially result in other conditions. That is why someone suffering from diabetes could have a heart attack.

Someone exercising to lose weight is actually making more bucks for his/her investment in terms of preventing heart attack and stroke.

High blood pressure

Incidents leading to a stroke have the tendency to increase the pressure in the blood reading. Blood pressure reading higher than 120/80 millimeter (mm Hg) could pose a risk of stroke if not controlled, or the root cause determined and treated. Please note that just because your blood pressure is greater than 120/80 mm Hg does not mean you are sick or should be worried. Your doctor is able to investigate and determine the root cause and decide if treatment is necessary. Self-medication is highly discouraged.

- High cholesterol (>200mg/dL or 5.2mMole per liter) is a risk factor for stroke.
- Cigarette smoking is a risk factor, not only for stroke, but also for heart attack.

Prior medical history or your lifestyle may contribute to the risk of stroke. For example: An overweight or obese patient has a high risk of stroke. A history of diabetes, heart failure, heart dysfunction are risk factors for stroke. Risky lifestyle, such as use of illicit drug such as cocaine and methamphetamines, certain birth control and genetic factors (family history of stroke) are known risk factors for stroke. Scientific study shows that the risk factor for stroke is more common in women than men with more death occurring in women than men.

There are several complications associated with stroke. The severity of these complications depends on the duration of the symptom before medical intervention. Stroke episodes literally deprive the brain of oxygen and important nutrients. The duration of oxygen or nutrient deprivation could lead to either death or disability. Complications from stroke includes loss of muscle movement or paralysis (total or partial), difficulty speaking or swallowing (lack of muscular coordination), memory loss or inability to think, reason or make sound judgment. Other forms of complications include emotional breakdown, depression, pain and loss of feeling and strange sensation in other parts of the body.

PREVENTION OF STROKE

We must take into account several factors that make healthy living a luxury for most people living in the developing country. However, knowledge of the symptoms, risk factors and preventive measures become a dangerous weapon of warfare against most common silent killer diseases. Understanding the risk factors associated with stroke is actually a big breakthrough in terms of prevention. Your problem is almost half solved by recognizing the potential sources.

Like most other cardiovascular diseases, adopting a healthy lifestyle is the best preventive measure for stroke. Most preventive measures for a stroke are the same as those recommended to help prevent a heart attack. Exercise and a healthy lifestyle that includes eating right will prevent stroke and other heart diseases. Unfortunately, some of the recommended lifestyles are difficult, if not impossible, to practice in some countries with acute poverty.

For example, in some rural areas, persons tend to do whatever necessary to stop hunger-by filling up their stomach with "anything in the name of food" and worry less about a balanced diet. As if that is not enough, the kind of alcoholic beverages sold in some poverty trodden regions of some developing countries are locally made "uncontrolled self-fed poison". As a result, the poor keep getting poorer where their health is concerned.

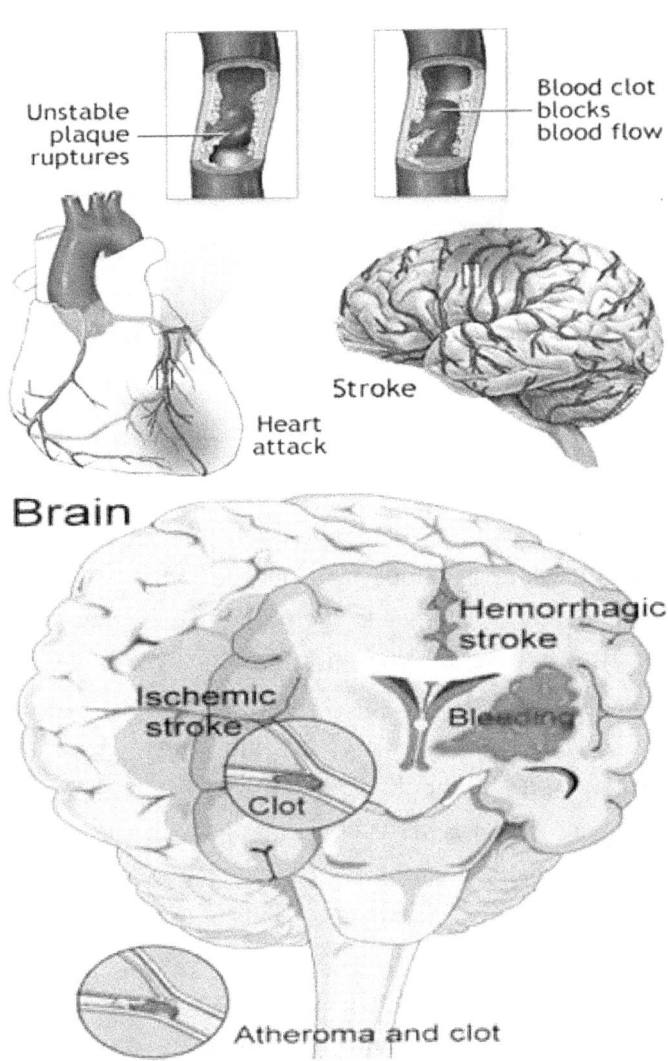

Blood Pressure	Systolic		Diastolic
Low Blood Pressure (hypotension)	50-90		35-60
Normal	Less than 120	and	Less than 80
High Normal (pre-hypertension)	120-139	or	80-89
High Blood Pressure (hypertension) stage 1	140-159	or	90-99
High Blood Pressure (hypertension) stage 2	160 or higher	or	100 or higher
High Blood Pressure (hypertension) stage 3/4	Higher than 180	or	Higher than 110

One of the controversial risk factors in regards to heart diseases is smoking. Despite what is known about it and warnings from the surgeon general, the addictive nature of this substance literally gives the consumer a deaf ear. However, study has shown that smoking cessation is by far the most preventive lifestyle for silent killer diseases. It bothers me however when people trade smoking with eating food as witnessed in most parts of poverty trodden areas of the developing countries. That is a recipe for destruction!

Finally, let us not neglect the danger this lifestyle poses on a smoker and their non-smoking family members who share the same home. If you are one of those persons who smoke at home, the smoke lingers longer in the house; the evidence is in the smell previewed hours and days after smoking. This results in a phenomenon called secondary inhalation of smoke, which also causes diseases such as asthma and cancer, another silent killer disease depending on the period of exposure. Smoking sounds a lot like self-poisoning.

CHAPTER 7
SILENT KILLER #4: EYE DISEASES

Eye diseases made it to the list of silent killers, unfortunately, due to its "chain reaction" effect on the victim. Some eye diseases are actually a residual effect of other silent killer diseases that manifest in a different form due to the part of body tissue, organ or artery that is affected. Like other silent killers diseases, most eye diseases present either deceptive symptoms or no symptoms at all making it difficult to be treated at onset. Also, because some people lack the basic knowledge and understanding of the symptoms of eye diseases, witchcraft is equally being cited as the culprit, giving the actual root cause enough time to fully incapacitate its host.

CATARACT EYE DISEASE

This is an eye condition that reduces the ability to see due to clouding of the eye lens. Just as difficult as it is driving with a foggy wind shield, so it is for someone with cataract eye disease. Seeing through a cloudy eye lenses is not only difficult, it is also stressful.

Cataract develops very slowly and in most cases does not disturb the eyesight at the onset of the

78

symptoms, making it difficult to detect without proper eye examination until it suddenly interferes with vision, even though the disease has gone undetected for a long time. For those who believe in witchcraft or who are used to citing witchcraft for any disease that appears suddenly, cataract meets their criterion. Like most silent killer diseases, if the symptoms are detected early, the use of corrective lenses could remedy the condition. However, if the disease developed to the stage where possible eye defect or vision impairment occurs, the patient might need a surgical procedure to remove the cataract. At the onset of cataract, the effect on the eyes is at its minimal but as the cataract grows, the eye lenses become cloudy and vision becomes blurred.

SYMPTOMS OF CATARACT

The following symptoms are associated with cataract:

- Blurred vision
- Sensitivity to light
- Fading or yellowing of colors
- Double vision in one eye
- Difficulty seeing at night

In the case of cataract and other silent killer diseases, preventive check-up with your doctor is the easiest way to detect and treat the disease. It is highly recommended that you get your eyes checked at least once every year. I know that for most people living in the developing countries, preventive check-ups without obvious onset of any disease is difficult to achieve for so many obvious reasons. However, I believe that this book will help change some of the perceptions regarding medicine, illness, preventive medicine and checkups. We cannot just "sit" and expect something to happen. I encourage you to start something, somewhere and somehow today no matter how small. We must continue trying until help arrives.

CAUSES OF CATARACT

Eye defects could be as a result of other medical conditions. In the case of cataract, it can be caused by other medical conditions such as diabetes, or trauma resulting from accident or surgery. Cataracts can also be as a result of genetic disorder inherited from parents. In most cases, cataracts can affect either of the eyes at a time, or both at same time. When cataract affects both eyes, it is possible that the cataract in one of the eyes has developed more than the other.

TYPES OF CATARACT

Cataract is classified based on how the affected eyes look. Cataract can affect the edges/corner of the eye lens (cortical cataract), the center of the eye lens (nuclear cataract) or the back of the eye lens (posterior cataract). Despite the part of the eye the cataract started, if it goes untreated after sometime, it will actually spread to other parts of the eye lens. In most cases, it leads to browning or yellowing of the eye lens resulting in problems with light glare and reduced vision.

There is another form of cataract called congenital cataracts. As the name implies, this is a form of cataract that some people are either born with or may have developed during the infant age. Infection during pregnancy could be a risk factor for congenital cataracts.

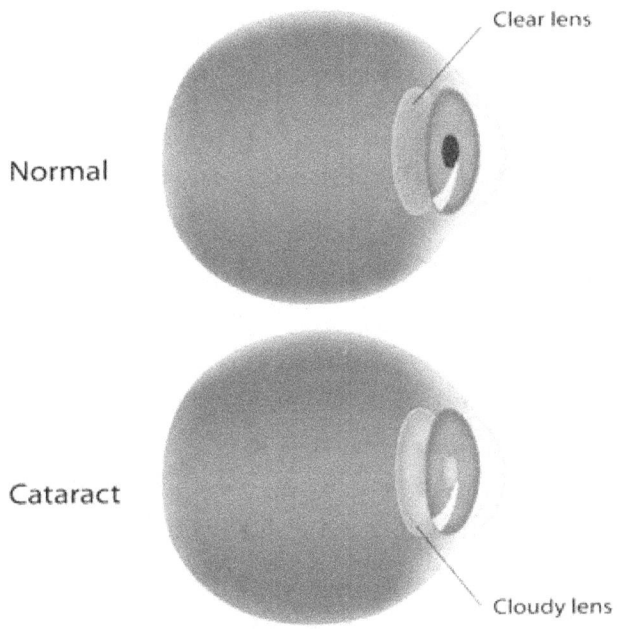

RISK FACTORS FOR CATARACTS

Some risk factors for cataracts include exposure to radiation, excessive exposure to sunlight (as in some sub-Saharan African countries), complications from other medical conditions such as diabetes and high blood pressure; complications from eye surgery, family history of cataract, obesity, unsafe lifestyle, excessive alcohol consumption and smoking. Sometimes cataract occurs as a combination of one or more risk factors.

PREVENTION OF CATARACT

Cataract is a treatable eye disease. Surgery has been proven as the most effective treatment for cataract, therefore, it is highly recommended that you discuss it with your eye doctor and find out when surgery would be necessary.

GLAUCOMA EYE DISEASE

Like most silent killer diseases, glaucoma is a dangerous eye disease that is capable of damaging the optical nerve resulting in partial or even permanent damage to your eye within a very short period. There are two known types of glaucoma diseases: open and closed-angle glaucoma. Glaucoma eye infection is associated with abnormally high eye pressure (just like the abnormal blood pressure for heart diseases). Also, like other silent killers, vision loss associated with glaucoma eye disease can go unnoticed for a long time until glaucoma complications sets in. In fact, some glaucoma diseases show no symptoms at all except noticeable gradual loss of vision.

Frequent eye checks are highly recommended, even without pre-existing eye conditions or abnormal conditions. In the case of glaucoma, early detection is the key to preventing further damage, especially to the optical nerves which could be due to the high eye (intraocular) pressure.

SYMPTOMS OF GLAUCOMA DISEASE

Symptoms of glaucoma eye diseases depend on the kind of glaucoma that infects the eyes. However, common known symptoms include; loss of vision (usually gradual), eye pain, blurred vision, and visual disturbances often in low light and halos around light. In my opinion, halos around light are the most disturbing symptom of glaucoma (personal experience).

CAUSES OF GLAUCOMA

In the diagnosis of glaucoma, tracing the root-cause can be challenging. Glaucoma is referred to as a primary condition when it is impossible to cite any other condition as the root cause of glaucoma; and a secondary condition when other known conditions could be cited as the root cause of the disease. Probable causes of glaucoma include prior injury to the eye, side effect from medication; complications from other eye conditions, inflammation and tumor.

Despite the root cause of glaucoma, early detection through comprehensive eye checks, especially for adults age 40 and older, is proven as an effective method of detection, treatment and prevention. If you forget everything you have learnt about symptoms of glaucoma, please do remember that whenever you experience severe headache or pain in the eyes, blurred vision, and halos around light, you may be suffering from glaucoma eye disease and you need to see your eye doctor immediately.

The high pressure associated with glaucoma is as a result of fluid buildup flowing in and out of the eye; which in some cases results in optical damage. For a normal eye, the fluid flows through and exits the eye through a drainage system formed between the cornea and iris. The eye drainage system is made up of the draining angle (formed between the cornea and iris) and drainage channels (meshwork) contained inside the angle, thereby maintaining a continuous fluid flow. However, in glaucoma infected eyes, it is possible that the natural drainage angle formed between the cornea and iris could remain open while the draining channels in the angle are partially blocked resulting in very slow drain (primary open-angle glaucoma).

In some cases, the iris may bulge forward causing the drainage angle formed between the iris and cornea to narrow significantly. In this scenario, flow of fluid through and exiting the eye is being significantly distorted, resulting in an abnormal increase in eye pressure (closed-angle glaucoma). Being born with narrowed drainage angle (shape formed between iris and cornea), unfortunately, is a risk factor for developing glaucoma. There is also another form of glaucoma referred to as "normal-tension glaucoma". As the name implies, a patient suffering from this kind of glaucoma unfortunately, maintain a "normal" eye pressure making it somewhat difficult to diagnose without other eye exam.

Although rare, glaucoma eye disease can occur at any point in someone's life; from birth to later age. Congenital glaucoma occurs when a baby is born with pre-existing glaucoma. Infantile glaucoma occurs when a child develops glaucoma within the first few years after birth.

RISK FACTORS FOR GLAUCOMA

One the reasons glaucoma eye diseases is on the list of silent killers among other factors is because the chronic form of glaucoma eye disease can destroy vision before any signs or symptoms are apparent. Risk factors for glaucoma include **Elevated internal eye pressure (intraocular pressure).** Your ophthalmologist or your optometrist should check your eye pressure whenever you visit for eye checkup. If your internal eye pressure is noted higher than normal during the checkup, then, you are at the risk of developing glaucoma. Please note that there are other factors that could lead to increase internal eye pressure, so not every incident of elevated eye pressure is attributed to glaucoma.

Age

Studies show that age is a risk factor for glaucoma eye diseases. Unfortunately you cannot control your ability to grow numerically old, but the knowledge of

85

risk factors associate with your numeric old age will help you maintain a healthy living. People older than 60 years of age are at high risk of most eye diseases, including glaucoma. You may be at higher risk of angle-closure glaucoma if you're older than age 40.

Ethnic background

Although we do not choose where we are born and to whom we are born, your ethnic background places you at high risk of some health problems. Unfortunately glaucoma eye disease is one of them. Study show that Africans or Black Americans older than 40 years old have a much higher risk of developing glaucoma than Caucasians (Oyibo) of the same age group. People of Asian descent have an increased risk of developing acute angle-closure glaucoma, while people of Japanese descent may be more likely to have normal-tension glaucoma.

Family history of glaucoma

Family history is a risk factor for all the silent killer disease we have examined so far. Knowing your family health history is not only beneficial knowledge, but will help you identify potential subjective risk factors and how to prevent them. Remember, "Prevention is better than cure"! Having a close family member with a history of eye glaucoma disease places you at risk of developing it.

Medical conditions

Most medical conditions are like a chemical chain reaction resulting into other conditions. Most silent killer provides a safe haven for other diseases invading your body. This is actually why it is important that we recognize these symptoms and treat them appropriately as soon as possible. Because silent killer diseases follow after one another in most instances, conspiracy theory capitalizes on that premise to cite witchcraft as the probable cause. Diabetes, heart diseases, high blood pressure and hypothyroidism are all risk factors for glaucoma eye disease.

COMPLICATIONS OF GLAUCOMA

If Glaucoma disease is left untreated, it has the tendency to lead to progressive vision loss: generate blind spots in your peripheral vision, tunnel vision and may result in total blindness.

TREATMENT OF GLAUCOMA

To treat glaucoma disease, your eye doctor usually focuses on lowering the pressure in your eye (intraocular pressure). In most cases, depending on the probable root cause and the damage, your eye doctors focuses on a process that will improve drainage of fluid in your eye or lower eye fluid production. Presently, there is no medical cure for glaucoma and or its associated damages, but treatment and regular checkups help prevent vision loss and further complications.

Eye-drops

One of the best known treatment or control of glaucoma disease is achieved using medicated eye drops. Remember your eyes might be so sensitive that the use of the wrong eye drop could cause more damage to your eyes. SELF-MEDICATION AND SELF PRESCRIPTION OF EYE DROPS IS HIGHLY DISCOURAGED. Your doctor should prescribe the eye drop for your condition based on the degree of damage and the type of glaucoma disease that affected your eyes. Your doctor may even prescribe more than one eye drop; in such case please make sure you ask your doctor how long to wait between applications and how long you will need to use the drop.

PREVENTION OF GLAUCOMA

Regular Eye Check

Annual preventive checkup with your primary care physician is a popular and affordable practice by many residents in developed countries. However, in Africa and other developing countries, preventive medicine is probably for the rich only. Families struggle to decide whether to take sick loved ones to the hospital or use the money to put food on the table for the entire family. Preventive checkup painfully becomes a luxury rather than necessity to some people living in developing countries.

There is no doubt that regular checkups (comprehensive eye exam) can help detect silent killer diseases in its early stages before further damage or other complications occur. As a general rule, it is highly recommended to have a comprehensive eye checkup every three to five years after age 40 and every year after age 60. However, if your doctor informs you that you are at a high risk of glaucoma or have been diagnosed with glaucoma; it is recommended to have your eyes checked every year. You may need more frequent screening if you have glaucoma risk factors. Your eye doctors should inform you on the frequency and the right eye screen.

Stick to the Treatment

In most cases, a few eye drops could relieve the glaucoma pain within a few days of the start of treatment. However, that does not mean that you should discontinue the treatment. It can be misleading sometimes, but it is necessary that you stick with the treatment plan recommended by your doctor. Normally, your doctor should gradually reduce the frequency of the eye drop use based on the pressure level and other symptoms.

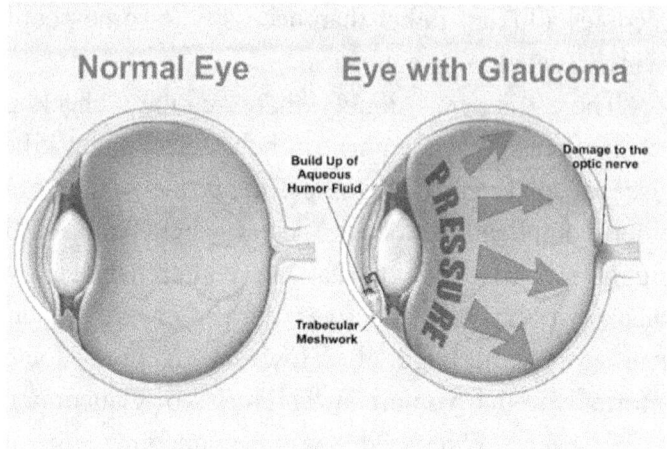

CHAPTER 8
SILENT KILLER #5: TUBERCULOSIS

The word Tuberculosis is derived from Latin word "tuberculum" which means small lump or pimple. This disease is caused by a bacterium known as "Mycobacterium tuberculosis" characterized by the infection of the lungs. Tuberculosis is a contagious airborne disease which means it can spread from one infected person to another person through the air in the form of microscopic droplets. It is commonly abbreviated as TB throughout the world.

This disease made the list of silent killers due to its ability to stay dormant or inactive in the body of the host for many years before the symptoms manifest. Normally, the host of the virus (Mycobacterium tuberculosis) is unable to identify it except during routine laboratory tests. Studies show that only ill adults are capable of spreading TB through coughing. Children can get infected with TB, but are not able to infect someone else. TB virus is very infectious and can affect many persons living in close proximity (same home) to each other within a short period of time.

SYMPTOMS OF TUBERCULOSIS

Studies show that the human lungs are the most susceptible site of attack for the virus mycobacterium tuberculosis. The commonly known signs and symptoms of Tuberculosis that attack the lungs includes but are not limited to:

- cough usually lasting between 2 or more weeks
- coughing up blood or sputum

Depending on the severity of the virus, other symptoms may include:

- chest pain, or pain with breathing.

Depending on the duration in the body, TB can also affect other parts of your body such as the kidneys, the spine or the brain.

Symptoms of TB may vary depending on the organ affected by the virus. Tuberculosis of the spine may result in back pain while, tuberculosis of the kidneys may produce blood in your urine. It is highly recommended that you go to your doctor for a medical test if you have a cough (associated with bloody sputum) that persists for more than 3 weeks to a month.

Another reason why this disease is considered deadly is partly due to the fact that adults affected by tuberculosis (even at its manifestation stage) do not feel sick other than the persistent cough.

Here is the problem, in some developing countries, people who are not able to pay for medical care can actually live with a persistent cough longer than 3 weeks as long as they are able to walk around and probably go to work. This is because even though your body may harbor the bacteria that cause tuberculosis; your immune system usually can prevent you from becoming sick. Due to the infectious nature of TB virus and the ability of the immune system to resist it as described above, this disease is considered very dangerous especially to the children who live in close proximity to the carrier.

For children and adolescents, commonly known symptoms of TB virus are fever, chills and night sweats, weight loss, infection of the bones and joints. It is quite unfortunate that the mortality rate in children due to TB virus is very high even when the disease is discovered early.

CLASSIFICATION OF TUBERCULOSIS

In general, Tuberculosis can be classified as either Latent or Active TB.

Latent TB

Tuberculosis is said to be in a latent state when a patient is infected by the virus, but the bacteria remains in your body in an inactive state causing no symptoms. Studies show that in a latent or inactive stage, TB infection is not contagious but has the tendency to become active in the future. Latent TB can be detected using laboratory test, and treatment is highly recommended even at the latent stage.

Active TB

TB is said to be in an active stage when the virus has active symptoms. In this stage, the victim is sick and capable of infecting other people. Depending on the part of the body infected, TB virus could become active in the first few weeks after infection of the host. Other symptoms of active TB include:

- Unintentional weight loss
- Fatigue
- Fever
- Loss of appetite
- Lethargic or fatigued body
- Shortness of breath

Tuberculosis virus can also be divided into Pulmonary and Extra-pulmonary Tuberculosis, based on the part of the body or organ affected:

- Laryngeal TB affects vocal chords and larynx
- Primary TB Pneumonia (Uncommon type with presence of Pneumonia, highly infectious)
- Pleurisy TB affects the Pleural space within the lungs
- Miliary Tuberculosis marked with the presence of small nodules throughout the lungs
- Cavitary TB marked with the formation of cavities throughout the lungs
- Adrenal TB affects smooth functioning of adrenal glands

- Lymphatic node-based TB primarily affects lymphatic nodes
- Meningitis TB affects meninges
- Renal TB greatly affects kidneys and reproductive organs
- Pericarditis TB halts badly smooth working of pericardium
- Osteal TB affects the bones

Important Notes

Please note that different diseases are capable of exhibiting the same kinds of symptoms, but your doctor can perform further tests to confirm suspected case of tuberculosis. TB virus can be contracted through sputum or inhaling droplets dispersed in the air when an infected person coughs or sneezes. You cannot acquire the disease by mere touching, hugging or shaking hands with the infected person. However, a person who stays or lives close to the infected person has a greater chance of being infected by the disease than other people. That is why it is recommended to test everyone living in the household once someone shows up positive with the TB virus.

While HIV does not lead to Tuberculosis infection, however, HIV virus weakens a person's immune system making it difficult for the body to fight the germ that causes TB.

CAUSES OF TUBERCULOSIS

Tuberculosis is an airborne disease - meaning that the bacteria can be spread from person to person through air. When an infected person with the untreated, active form of tuberculosis coughs, speaks, sneezes or spits, some microscopic droplets are released into the air. The microscopic droplets contain the TB-causing germs which can cause the virus when a healthy person inhales it. The good news is that with appropriate treatment for about 2 weeks, active and contagious TB can be rendered inactive.

Recent scientific studies have shown that some strains of tuberculosis are drug-resistant. Drug-resistant strains of tuberculosis emerge when an antibiotic fails to kill all of the bacteria it targets. The surviving bacteria become resistant to that particular drug and frequently other antibiotics as well. Eradication of active tuberculosis requires that the patient take several types of medications for many months, failure to do so could result in the development of a drug resistance strain.

COMPLICATIONS RELATED TO TUBERCULOSIS

Like other silent killer diseases, if tuberculosis is left untreated it may result in great damage to your body or even lead to death. For example, Osteal TB greatly affects the health of your bones while renal TB can cause real damage to your kidneys or other reproductive organs if undetected and untreated.

Untreated active disease can affect your lungs or spread to other parts of the body through your bloodstream. Some complications related to TB include;

- spinal pain and joint destruction, including the rib region;
- brain meningitis - fatal swelling of the membranes that covers your brain and spinal cord;
- impairment of the liver or kidneys.

Finally, when tuberculosis is left untreated, it may result in inflammation of the heart region resulting in heart malfunction (cardiac tamponade).

RISK FACTORS FOR TUBERCULOSIS

People at high risk for this infection can broadly be categorized into two main categories:

- Those who have recently been diagnosed with TB
- Those with weak immune system.

As stated earlier, other medical conditions such as HIV could weaken someone's immune system and make them susceptible to tuberculosis.

- You are at the high risk of tuberculosis if:
- You live in a "confined" space with someone who has TB.
- Consume contaminated food or water.
- Use illegal drugs

There are different factors that could contribute to developing tuberculosis. Some of the factors may increase the risk of acquiring tuberculosis more than others.

Immune Deficient Conditions

Naturally, your body is wired to fight foreign bodies such as diseases (tuberculosis virus included) if your immune system is active (strong). However, some medical conditions can result in "immune deficient syndrome" making your body unable to fight or defend itself." Studies also show that some medical conditions or drug use could render your immune system inactive or weak. Medical conditions such as:

- HIV/AIDS
- Diabetes
- Certain cancers
- Transplant Drugs
- Malnutrition

Also, some people fail to care for their body due to poverty or lack of knowledge of hygiene. A majority of the persons living in developing countries do not have the luxury of caring for or choosing what to eat and when to eat it. For some people all they care about is to literally fill up their stomach regardless of the nutritional composition of the food item. Unfortunately, not everything we eat adds value to our body but everything we eat affects our body in different forms. The body system absorbs the nutrient

98

or poison from the food we eat resulting in an improved immune system or deficient immune condition.

In most parts of the developing countries, people drink all kinds of herbs either as part of alcoholic drinks or for curative purposes. While some of the substances are intoxicating (which explains affinity by most of the locals) the substance may be dangerous to the immune system making the body susceptible and easily prone to disease.

TREATMENT AND PREVENTION OF TUBERCULOSIS

This book is basically about prevention, especially owing to the level of poverty and financial constrain in most developing countries, prevention will surely be better than cure. For example, getting tested and possibly treated for cough or similar symptoms that have lasted more than one month will help rule out or confirm the presence of a disease virus.

For folks who have already been diagnosed with tuberculosis, keeping up with the enormous number of medications prescribed for treatment of tuberculosis might be challenging. However, it is very necessary that the medication regiment be maintained until your health provider confirms that you are completely free of the virus. In most cases, the medication or treatment could last between 6 to 12 months if the patient follows their doctor's prescription. Failure to do so could result in re-emergence of the disease.

The most commonly used diagnostic tool for tuberculosis is a simple skin test. A small amount of a substance called PPD tuberculin is injected just below the skin of your inside forearm. A medical technician checks for swelling at (the site where the PPD was injected) within 48 to 72 hours. A hard, raised red bump means you are positive and there's a possibility you may have been infected by TB causing virus. The size of the bump is a factor in determining the validity of the test.

Please note: if you received the BCG vaccine as a child, there is a very high chance of your PPD test being positive. In that case, your doctor is likely to order a chest X-ray to rule out possible tuberculosis infection. A chest x-ray for positive tuberculosis virus infection will show white spots or significant changes in the lungs where your immune system has walled off the TB bacteria.

Another way to test, confirm and prevent tuberculosis virus is by testing the mucus that comes up when the patient coughs (sputum). Remember, TB virus may remain in a latent status for months before manifesting as a highly infectious disease. This is another reason why testing every relative of a patient with active TB is highly recommended and important as well.

The following basics must be followed to prevent the spread of tuberculosis:

100

- Don't spend long periods of time with or around a person infected by TB.
- Use protective face masks when entering the tuberculosis patients room or environment
- To ensure safety of others, always place your hands in front of your mouth while sneezing or coughing.

At this point, you already know the difference between latent and active tuberculosis. During the preventive testing for tuberculosis, your doctor will check you for both latent and active tuberculosis. Although only the active tuberculosis is contagious, if your test result shows positive for latent TB, you doctor will prescribe medication to treat you for tuberculosis.

If your test results show positive for active (contagious) tuberculosis, you should take all necessary precaution not only to treat yourself, but to ensure your family and friends are safe from risk of being infected. To ensure your friends and family are safe from the dangers of contracting tuberculosis, you should avoid sleeping in a room with other people, going to work or other public places with the possibility of infecting people. Ensure that the room where you stay is grossly ventilated to help reduce the condensation of droplet in the surrounding air. When you are around people (family friends or coworkers) wearing surgical mask will help prevent discharge of droplets into the air.

At a certain age, infants in most countries are vaccinated against tuberculosis using the bacille Calmette-Guerin (BCG) vaccine. This vaccine will help protect the child and reduce the risk of severe tuberculosis infection. Meanwhile, the person may still contract tuberculosis with increased risk factors during the course of life.

Dr. Eugene C. Uche

CHAPTER 9
SILENT KILLER #6: DIARRHEA

Diarrhea can be defined as an illness where one passes watery or loose stools frequently, often more than 3 times in a day. According to world health organization, diarrhea kills more than 4 million children every year (more than 10,000 per day). Unfortunately, diarrhea as a silent killer can strike anyone at any point in time and can last from a few days to months.

Diarrhea could be triggered by infections, intestinal disorders and certain medical conditions. According to the National Institutes of Health, the average adult can expect about four bouts of acute diarrhea per year. Children in the United States average 7 to 15 episodes of diarrhea by age 5. The statistics is greater for children in the developing countries and rural areas with poor sanitary facilities.

CLASSES OF DIARRHEA

I will classify diarrhea as acute or chronic depending on the severity and duration of the symptoms. Diarrhea can be referred to as acute if the symptoms disappeared within 14 days; but chronic diarrhea could last between 2 to 4 weeks. Acute

103

diarrhea is typically due to a viral or bacterial infection, while chronic diarrhea is more likely to be caused by underlying medical conditions.

In reference to root causes, Diarrhea can be classified as osmotic and exudative.

Osmotic Diarrhea

Diarrhea is said to be osmotic (derived from osmosis) when, for example, excess sugar or salt in a drink draws water from the body to the bowels. Some common examples may include 'chewing gum' or 'dietetic candy' where sorbitol, a sugar substitute, does not get absorbed by the body; but rather draws water into the bowel. Sometimes due to several other factors such as the presence of disease or certain drugs, the body increases release of water into the bowel resulting in diarrhea.

Exudative Diarrhea

Exudative diarrhea refers to diarrhea resulting from inflammatory diseases of the bowel caused by some kind of infection or food poisoning. In most cases of exudative diarrhea, blood in stool sample is evident.

SYMPTOMS OF DIARRHEA

Symptoms of diarrhea varies from more common loose or watery stool, bloating, cramps, urgent bowel movements, vomiting and feeling nausea to more complicated symptoms such as; evidence of pus and

104

blood in the stool, often referred to as Dysentry, undigested food in the stool, weight loss and high fever.

The good news here is that the majority of these symptoms produces obvious changes to your system and could be recognized as soon as they present themselves. However, it is your responsibility to seek for medical attention once the symptoms mature from acute to chronic or you notice sudden increase in the severity of the associated symptoms. For example, diarrhea resulting from food poisoning is likely to progress in severity faster than diarrhea resulting from consumption of sugary or salty substances.

CAUSES OF DIARRHEA

The most common known cause of diarrhea is viral infection especially to the gut. Other causes include:

- Bacterial infection or infection from several organism, or parasites.
- An allergy to some foods.
- Complications from other diseases such as-diabetes, certain cancers, some intestinal diseases including crohn's disease and ulcerative cohtis.
- In most cases, some food items may be mal-absorbed into the body or may upset the digestive system resulting in diarrhea "upset stomach".

- Abuse of laxatives and/ or alcohol can result in diarrhea.
- Some medications including radiation, surgery of the digestive track, and certain drugs.
- Environmental conditions (lack of hygiene)

In general, diarrhea is known to occur as a result of gastroenteritis diseases of the digestive track such as salmonella bacteria, shigella, and E. coli; viruses like rotavirus, cytomegalovirus, and viral hepatitis; parasites such as cryptosporidium, Giardia lamblia, and Entamoeba histolytica.

Other possible causes of diarrhea include:

- Eating undercooked meats or unrefrigerated food
- Drinking from or swimming in contaminated water.

In most parts of the developing countries, sewer management is of great environmental concern and can be cited as a source of diarrheal diseases. Diarrhea is infectious and must be handled with care especially when caring for a patient or loved one that is having diarrhea.

Other than being infected by diarrheal bacterial, sensitivity to certain foods such as dairy products and artificial sweeteners could cause diarrhea. Also, adverse effects of some medications may include diarrhea. As a result, if you experience changes in your stool or frequency of "going" make sure you inform your doctor of the changes. Locally, some people

106

consume herbs and mixture of substance when they "feel heavy" to induce diarrhea.

One big advice in the event of diarrhea; avoid sugary and fatty food. Unfortunately millions of the people living in developing countries do not have much to eat; nor do they have the luxury to choose the kind of food to avoid. The best strategy will be to avoid any condition that may result to diarrhea. Ensure you drink plenty of fluids but avoid alcohol beverages and caffeine. Alcohol and caffeinated beverages in a diarrheal condition is a recipe for dehydration. The key to surviving diarrhea is to stay hydrated as much as possible. Possible signs of dehydration during diarrhea include dry mouth or dry skin, fatigue, amount of urine and deep coloration of urine.

PREVENTION OF DIARRHEA

Diarrhea is an infectious disease that is able to spread from one human to another. It is therefore very important to take necessary precautions to avoid direct contact with someone already having symptoms of diarrhea. The following safe precaution must be taken to ensure diarrheal disease is contained and to avoid person to person spread:

- Hand hygiene! Always wash your hand frequently before eating, after eating and after using the bathroom.

- Ensure the environment where you process your food (raw food including meat) is clean and sanitized.

- Ensure you thoroughly wash all raw food, fruits and vegetable before cooking (hot water washing recommended). Vegetables and fruits consumed raw such as Mango, Apples, Oranges, and Berries etc. must be thoroughly washed. It is possible that the vegetable or fruit has come in contact with animal feces.

- Unfortunately, I have to inform you that eating food from the roadside vendor (Mama-Put) is a very risky act. The mama-put environment in most of the countries I have visited is a recipe for diarrhea disaster and food poisoning.

- You must pay close attention to the drinking water source; this is the most common source of diarrhea.

- If you are having diarrhea, make sure you avoid drinking milk or milk products, but rather drink plenty of water and electrolytic drinks.

- It is recommended that you follow the "BRAT" DIET plan (Bananas, Rice, Applesauce, and Toast). BRAT is popular diet blend that consists of foods that are low in fiber. Unfortunately, for most people in poverty trodden region of the world, these food items are luxury.

- If you are having diarrhea, take a break from work and other strenuous activities.
- If you are pregnant and having symptoms of diarrhea, please call your doctor as soon as possible.
- For both adults and children, it is recommended that they drink plenty of fluids to stay hydrated at all times. For example, special electrolyte Pedialyte is formulated to replenish body nutrient in children having diarrhea symptoms.
- Exclusive breastfeeding of children for at least six months is important for a child's development and it strengthens their immune system.
- The role of hygiene in preventing diarrhea cannot be over-emphasized. Hygiene helps much in the prevention of diarrhea, especially for children who are vulnerable to dirt.

TREATMENT OF DIARRHEA

In general, diarrhea is not such a deadly medical condition compared to other silent killers we have discussed so far. However, if left untreated or allowed longer than necessary, it may lead to other complications including death. Diarrhea is very common both in developed and developing country. One of the dangerous complications associated with diarrhea is loss of fluid.

Oral rehydration solution, ORS, is the most popular and effective method for treating diarrhea because of its hydration capability. Unfortunately, some people may vomit after drinking ORS, therefore it is recommended to drink it slowly and in bits.

Please avoid sugary drinks such as soda especially with children as they increase the rate of dehydration during diarrhea. Continue normal feeding routine for your child even if they are vomiting or throwing up after meal. Breastfeeding is highly encouraged for children that are still breastfeeding. Please note that ORS does not negate the need for medical professionals. If symptoms persist, you need to call or visit your doctor immediately. The ORS is necessary to prevent and treat dehydration by replacing the fluid and minerals that are lost during the diarrhea and vomiting. Remember, what kills diarrhea patients is the dehydration from diarrhea not the diarrhea.

How to Prepare ORS at Home

The following steps are used to prepare ORS at home. The following ingredients are required;
- Real Salt
- Potassium Chloride Salt
- Baking Soda
- Granulated Sugar

Measure and mix the ingredients listed above together using the combination below: ¼ -teaspoon real salt, ¼-teaspoon potassium chloride salt, ¼-

teaspoon baking soda and 2 ½- tablespoon granulated sugar. Add 4-cups of water to this mixture making sure the mixture is as accurate as possible. If the concentration is not right, the patient may become sicker.

Finally, mix the solution very well using a spoon to stir. The good news is, you now have your ORS.

Treatment of Diarrhea using ORS

The World Health Organization (WHO) recommended the steps below for preparing Oral Rehydration Solution to ensure it is safe and hygienic. To ensure that the solution is aseptic, WHO recommends you use about 1 liter (32 OZ) of water that has been boiled for at least 1 minute, covered and cooled. You can use the already mixed ORS pack (if available) or you can locally prepare ORS in the comfort of your home. 1 ORS pack to1 liter (32 oz).

Depending on where you live, the ORS package may be obtained from the pharmacy or health centers. To ensure a safe and lifesaving procedure for preparing ORS and treating diarrhea, follow the exact rules from WHO. Same treatment principles apply to both children and adults.

STEP 1: Give the Child More Fluids than Usual to Prevent Dehydration:

Use recommended home fluids! ORS solution is the best for all ages as it is next to breast milk. Purified plain water is also good and may be used for all ages, however plain water does not replace the salts that are lost in the stool. Ensure that the ORS is being given with a cup and spoon. Never use baby bottles. Baby bottles are very difficult to keep clean and can contain deadly germs.

For Children over 6 months old, you may, in addition, use food-based fluids that the child has had before. Many countries have designated recommended home fluids. Wherever possible, these should include at least one fluid that normally contains salt. Plain clean water should also be given.

Unsuitable fluids

A few fluids are potentially dangerous and should be avoided during diarrhea. Some examples are: Commercial soda and other carbonated beverages, commercial fruit juices, Sweetened tea, Coffee, Some medicinal teas or infusions.

Suitable fluids

Most fluids that a child normally takes can be used. It is helpful to divide suitable fluids into two groups:

Fluids that normally contain salt, such as: ORS solution, salted drinks (e.g. salted rice water or a salted yogurt drink), vegetable or chicken soup with salt.

Fluids that do not contain salt, such as: Plain safe water, Water in which a cereal has been cooked (e.g. unsalted rice water), unsalted soup, yogurt drinks without salt, green coconut water. weak tea (unsweetened), unsweetened fresh fruit juice.

Give as much of these fluids as the child will take. Continue giving more of these fluids until the diarrhea stops.

STEP 2: Give supplemental zinc (Up to 6 months of age: 10mg every day for 14 days. Six months or more: 20mg every day for 14 days.)

Zinc can be given as syrup or as dispersible tablets, whichever formulation is available and affordable. By giving zinc as soon as diarrhea starts, the duration and severity of the episode as well as the risk of dehydration will be reduced. By continuing zinc supplementation for 10 to 14 days, the zinc lost during diarrhea is fully replaced and the risk of the child having new episodes of diarrhea in the following 2 to 3 months is reduced.

STEP 3: Give the Child Plenty of Food to Prevent Under-nutrition.

Increase the frequency of breast-feeding. Breast feeding is always what is most important both for prevention and treatment of diarrhea. If the child is not breast-fed, give the usual cow's milk in a cup. However, if the cow's milk seem to make the diarrhea worse, you may have to temporarily change to a lactose free formula such as soy.

If the child is six months or older you may continue to give the following foods, if the child has had them before:

- cereal or another starchy food mixed, with milk or pulses (peas, beans, lentils, and similar

plants having pods), vegetables, meat, fish or egg.
- fresh fruit or mashed banana or green coconut water to provide potassium.
- freshly prepared foods; cook and grind food well to help digestion.

Encourage the child to eat:
- Frequent, small feedings are tolerated well than less frequent, large ones.
- Give the same food after diarrhea stops, and give an extra meal each day for two weeks.

While the person is having diarrhea: Their body needs some sugar and ORS contains exactly the right amount. However, do not give foods high in sugars (Sodas and sweetened drinks such as tea, coffee which also contain stimulants or other drinks or to which sugar has been added)--These draw water into the intestine and make the diarrhea worse. With diarrhea, you also have to be careful with commercial fruit juices. For nearly all other illnesses, fruit juices are excellent.

STEP 4: Take the person with diarrhea to the health provider if she/he develops any of the following:
- does not get better in three days
- more watery stools
- develops a fever or looks sicker
- repeated vomiting
- blood in the stool

114

- eating or drinking poorly
- becomes very thirsty
- Seems to be getting dehydrated.

How to Give ORS

- Begin with a tablespoon every 1–2 minutes for a child under 2 years.
- Give frequent sips from a cup for older children.
- The amount can be gradually increased as long as there is no vomiting.
- If the child vomits, wait 5-10 minutes. Then give the solution more slowly (for example, a spoonful every 2–3 minutes and gradually increase as tolerated).
- If diarrhea continues after the ORS packets are used up, give other fluids as described

CHAPTER 10
SILENT KILLER # 7: TETANUS

Tetanus is a bacterial disease that affects the nervous system, resulting in painful muscle contractions, especially the jaw and neck muscles. The bacteria that cause the disease Tetanus is known as bacterium *Clostridium tetani*. In an episode of muscle spasm, the jaw is "locked" as a result some people refer to this disease as "lockjaw." This disease made the list of silent killer disease for the following reasons:

- No hospital lab tests exist that can confirm tetanus
- Your doctor can only rely on examination and manifestation of certain signs and symptoms to confirm the disease
- Tetanus requires immediate treatment with human tetanus immune globulin (TIG) (or equine antitoxin) which in most cases is not available depending on your location
- Tetanus has no cure but there are drugs to control muscle spasms
- Muscle spasms are very painful

- There is an abundance of its spores in our environment especially in the developing countries with poor environmental conditions.
- Tetanus disease grows in dirty wounds and in most cases in the umbilical cord, if the cord is cut with a non-sterile instrument.

In most parts of the developing countries, women still deliver their babies at home or at a local herbalist with no knowledge of infection control. The tendency of infection either from dirty wounds or unsterilized equipment used in child delivery in this part of the world is alarmingly high. Tetanus is a life threatening disease because of its ability to distort breathing.

According to the World Health Organization report, more than a million cases of tetanus occur every year worldwide and majority of these cases reported are in developing countries. Although immunization has tremendously reduced the rate of infection recorded all over the world, awareness and preventive measures (understanding risk factors and symptoms) are necessary to ensure the incident rate is reduced.

SYMPTOMS OF TETANUS INFECTION

Like most silent killer diseases, signs and symptoms of tetanus infection may appear unnoticed and unexpected. In most cases, injuries you choose to "tough out" could be infected with tetanus in a few days or several weeks after. Studies show that tetanus bacteria have an incubation period of 7-10 days before the symptom manifests.

Signs and symptoms associated with tetanus infection include:

- Muscle spasms and stiffness especially in the jaw, neck and abdominal muscles
- Difficulty swallowing
- Painful body spasms lasting for several minutes, typically triggered by minor occurrences, such as a draft, loud noise, physical touch or light
- Fever (in some cases)
- Sweating
- May also result in elevated blood pressure and rapid heart rate.

CAUSES OF TETANUS

As sated earlier, the bacteria that causes the disease Tetanus is known as bacterium *Clostridium tetani*. This bacterium is actually found in soil, dust and animal feces. Unfortunately all the possible hosts of bacterium *Clostridium tetani* listed above are part of our immediate environment. That means we live and integrate with these bacteria every moment of our lives. At any point in time these bacteria can find its way into the human body (usually through deep flesh wound) the spores of the bacteria produces a powerful toxin, called tetanospasmin. The toxin directly attacks the nerves that control your muscles (through the motor neuron) causing muscle stiffness and spasms.

Another possible point of contact with the body is the use of unsterilized equipment in dressing wounds or cutting an umbilical cord during delivery (scary but it happens very often). In most rural villages, the locals tend to neglect the danger of tetanus when they have a cut, either because they are ignorant of the bacteria or they lack knowledge of the risk factors.

RISK FACTORS OF TETANUS

In order for tetanus causing bacteria to survive in the host's body, certain factors must be present. There are a whole laundry lists of risk factors for tetanus disease including;

- Lack of immunization
- Inadequate immunization (it is required that you also take booster shots against tetanus)
- Lack of care for deep cut injury
- Presence of other infectious bacteria
- Infected newborn's umbilical stump from unsterilized equipment.
- Neonatal tetanus maybe as a result of inadequately immunized mothers
- People of all ages can get tetanus
- Tetanus is common and serious in newborn babies (neonatal tetanus).
- Swelling around the injury

- Puncture wounds — including from splinters, body piercings, tattoos, injection drugs (especially if the instrument is not well sterilized)
- Gunshot wounds (if not treated immediately)
- Compound fractures
- Burns
- Surgical wounds
- Injection drug use
- Animal bites

COMPLICATIONS OF TETANUS

When the bacteria (tetanus) invades the body, the spore releases toxins which are capable of "bonding" with the nerves. Unfortunately, it is currently impossible to remove the toxin from the nerve ending once bonded. Until the infected nerve regenerates, the patient (victim) will not be able to recover. Nerve regeneration could take several months depending on other medical conditions and factors.

Tetanus infection is very painful due to the effect of the disease on the muscle such as spasm, jaw lock, etc. Health complications associated with tetanus infection ranges from impairment to loss of life. Victims of tetanus infection suffer from several episodes of muscle spasms per day; depending on the severity of spasm, the victim may suffer broken bones and spine, damage to the brain and mental defect. In most cases, the severity of the muscle spasm may lead to difficulty breathing, leading to respiratory system malfunction, cardiac arrest, pneumonia and possibly death.

PREVENTION OF TETANUS INFECTION

So far, we have learned that to be able to survive some of the complications of tetanus infection, medical attention need to be provided immediately as the signs and symptoms manifest. Meanwhile, for some living in the developing countries (rural areas) medical care is just one of the items on the bucket list. Some of the patients are left to die because the people are ignorant of the root cause. In some areas, they could easily attribute muscle spasm as a demonic manifestation confirming their suspicion that the patient is probably under some witch spell.

The only way to survive where there is no doctor is to stay healthy.

In the case of tetanus infection, the best prevention is immunization against the disease. People who were not immunized are at a higher risk of contracting the disease. Immunization against tetanus must be followed by "booster shot" about 10 years later. The vaccine used to protect against tetanus infection is called DTaP (Diphtheria, Tetanus toxide, and Acellular Pertussis). The DTaP vaccine consists of a series of five shots given at ages:

- 2 months
- 4 months

- 6 months
- 15 to 18 months
- 4 to 6 years

TREATMENT, LIFESTYLE CHANGES AND REMEDIES

Remember, there is no scientific proven treatment for tetanus infection. However, possible treatment consists of wound care and medications to ease symptoms such as spasms. With time, the infected nerve regenerates and the symptoms go away. If the source of tetanus is an open deep cut, cleaning the wound with disinfectant is essential to inhibit growth of the tetanus spores.

For people in areas with medical support, treatment that focuses on respiratory support in an intensive care setting is required, since the disease often results in shallow to difficulty breathing. In most cases support by ventilator may be needed. Unfortunately, in most part of the developing countries, hospitals are not equipped to provide such a high level of respiratory care. For people living in those areas, prevention is your best line of defense.

Most people living in the developing countries with medical facilities do not have medical insurance, which means that you pay out of pocket for every medical service provided to you. As if that was not enough, some people (unfortunately) are put in a position where they have to choose between feeding and healthcare. This increases the risk factor for silent killer diseases such as tetanus infection. Self-medication and self-treatment become the acceptable norm in a situation like this since the people cannot afford the cost of medical care in the hospital or health center. For example, self-treated puncture wounds or other deep cuts may turn to dirty or infected wounds and increase the risk of tetanus infection because the equipment or product used in cleaning the wound is dirty.

Where possible, avoid treating the wound yourself without having a trained doctor examine it, clean it, and apply antibiotic if needed. In some instances, your doctor will give you a booster shot of the tetanus toxoid vaccine to inhibit growth of tetanus spore. To prevent the chance of tetanus infection, the following steps are recommended when you have a cut (especially minor wound):

- **Stop the Bleeding**

If the wound is bleeding, the first recommended therapy to help stop the bleeding is to apply direct pressure to control the bleeding. However, you should be careful not to introduce dirt in this process since the wound is exposed.

- **Keep it Clean and Covered**

Applying pressure on the wound will stop the bleeding; however, the duration of pressure may vary depending on the severity of the cut, prior medical conditions and genetic make-up. After the bleeding has stopped, rinse the wound thoroughly with clean running water, soap and a clean washcloth (towel). The use of a saline solution is recommended (if available). Exposing the wound to the air may speed healing, however bandages can help keep the wound clean and keep harmful bacteria out. If the wound is not clean, the bandage will actually keep the bacteria in causing infection. It is recommended that you change the soiled bandage (dressing) daily to reduce the risk of infection.

- **Apply Antibiotic**

Cleaning the wound is the first step to protecting against tetanus. However, it is recommended that you apply a thin layer of an antibiotic cream or ointment. Depending on your location antibiotics such as Neosporin and Polysporin could be purchased over the counter. There are hundreds of other antibiotic creams and ointments in different countries but a majority of them contain same active ingredient that is capable of preventing tetanus spore growth and infection.

Conclusion

Numerous scientific research have shown that human behavior and belief play an important role in the spread and control of infectious diseases, and understanding the influence of ideology and belief system on the spread of diseases can be the key to improving control efforts. One thing both the rich and the poor will agree on with much controversy is that we all need good health. Unfortunately, the definition of good health and acceptable approach to meeting that goal remains a problem.

As I literally watch the deadly, merciless killer, Ebola Virus Disease (EVD) epidemics unfold and devastate some cities and countries in Africa, I could not agree more that ignorance is the father of all mishaps. Between March and August 2014, this Ebola virus affected more than 2200 people in about 4 nations in Africa. There were many conspiracy theories; very normal in a situation like this, but the incidence rate of this killer disease unconditionally caught my attention.

The incident rate of Ebola Virus disease in most African nations is a clear evidence of what happens when the knowledge of symptoms and preventive measures of a particular disease is missing in action. Also, the rate of spread of the Ebola killer disease depicts the gap between what we believe and what we know. Unfortunately the Ebola Virus Epidemic was not discussed in this series due to uncertainties surrounding the diagnosis, treatment and prevention of the diseases. Another lesson drawn from the ongoing effort to control or contain this killer disease in most poverty trodden cities of Africa is the conflict between human behavior, culture and belief.

According to the AFP news, a health official in Sierra Leone revealed that the outbreak need never have spread from Guinea, except for an herbalist in the remote eastern border village of Sokoma, who "...was claiming to have powers to heal Ebola. As a result, patients from Guinea infected with Ebola were crossing into Sierra Leone for treatment." Suddenly, "She got infected and died. During her funeral, women around the other towns got infected." The herbalist's mourners fanned out across the rolling hills of the Kissi tribal chiefdoms, starting a chain reaction of infections, deaths, funerals and more infections. A worrying outbreak turned into a major epidemic when the virus finally hit Kenema city.

Before now, most people are of the belief that what you did not know will not harm you. Numerous incidents, especially disease outbreaks, have not only proven that belief to be myth but has shown that a lack of knowledge of potential silent killers will steal, kill and equally destroy.

The Ignoramus series 1 - Understanding the Silent Killer Disease was designed to shed light on the burden culture and belief has placed on the human race, especially when it comes to health belief. Undoubtedly, global epidemics of our time have proven that knowledge of symptoms and disease risk factor is the key to establishing trust, share understanding and aid our quest to know more, especially among the population deeply rooted in the belief of witchcraft and other conspiracy theories.

I read a story of a young medical student who volunteered to help in Haiti right after the devastation caused by the 2010 earthquake. Like most foreigners in some of the developing nations, he was surprised on how most common mistakes could lead to a wide spread disease outbreak. Haiti experienced a great outbreak of Cholera (a killer disease) as an after effect of the earthquake. Despite the fact that a network of cholera treatment centers and stabilization centers were established in coordination with the Ministry of Health, the cholera outbreak took the health workers by surprise as a result of human behavior fueled by their belief. Unfortunately, between October 20 and November 9, Partners in Health recorded 7159 cases of severe cholera. The problem is that some aid workers who travel to most of the disease trodden regions probably thought that the people they have come to assist would literally roll out the red carpet for them. Although in most cases they did receive a royal welcome in some areas, that was not always the experience. There were significant differences between what the people believed and what they were proposing.

To a westerner, the instruction "do not touch your loved one" when suspected of some symptoms that could be of a deadly infectious disease may be received as a preventive measure, but in some cultures and beliefs, that is total dissertation especially when the person infected is the spouse. Understanding and considering some of the cultural and religious belief in the developing countries will foster understanding and trust among the medical personnel and the members of the community.

It is possible that the alleged incident in Kennema Sierrra Leone that led to the spread of Ebola in that region was possible because of the pre-existing trust among the members of the community's acclaimed traditional healer. It is possible, if not obvious, that the reason witchcraft is cited as the cause of death whenever someone dies of any of the symptoms of silent killer diseases is because the people do not know better. How can you miss something you've never known? If all they grew up to know and believe is that witchcraft is responsible for sudden death, it will take another effort to make them understand that there is more to that theory than they will ever know.

Knowledge is an ever required ingredient for human growth and metamorphosis, and we tend to hang on to what we know until proven otherwise.

This book is designed as an intervention aimed at changing such behaviors and largely to encourage people to reflect on their behaviors, their beliefs and based on what they now know in regards to signs, symptoms and risk factors of silent killer diseases. In order to effectively address these issues, both "the people" and public health workers must be empowered through health education, knowledge impact of cultural differences and how those differences affect treatment and other preventive health decisions. One important step we must take toward strengthening our citizenry in developing countries is to develop a clear framework that will aid in the identification of symptoms, preventative measures, diagnosis and treatment of disease (where possible).

The burdens of health affect both the rich and the poor. For example, the recent Ebola disease outbreak has killed several medical professionals (that the poor nations are already in shortage of them) who were providing care for the patients. Unfortunately, we live in a time when people are quick to blame one another or criticize the government for either not doing enough or not doing anything at all. Although it is the responsibility of every government to provide both security and healthcare for their citizenry, not doing anything at all, because our government is not living up to our expectation, is a deadly recipe.

I believe that the burden of health care and health promotion among the people in our communities must be treated as a joint venture between the people, the religious community and the government. Pursuing the goal of improved health literacy and to change the status quo will require active collaboration between health workers/educators, religious leaders and the government. Our religious leaders will have to play the role of health educators and help implement programs that are informative, and help their members to develop confidence to ask and act on the right information where their health is concerned. Government and religious organizations must also enter into strategic partnership to help promote health education, especially those that assist the people to recognize the signs and symptoms of silent killer diseases.

Growing up in Nigeria in the 80's, there used to be Health centers (government-sponsored local clinics) in different cities. Unfortunately, those clinics have gradually been shut down for lack of funding from the government. I usually don't like to comment on the system of government as I know there could be other constructive reasons why those health centers were shut down. However, you cannot afford to take the only hope of preventive care away from the communities without a viable alternative for emergency health care. In some developing countries, it could take hours or even days (in some parts of Kenya) to get to the nearest "hospital-like" facility. Unfortunately, most of the people living in those remote areas are farmers who are prone to injuries that will require medical care and immunization against tetanus.

In regards to funding the health clinic, a well-designed community health initiative would reduce the cost requirement with less financial burdens on the government. In fact, in some countries university graduates are mandated to complete a one year national service. This could be an opportunity to equip the health centers with skilled medical professionals all year round. The good news here is that some of the young graduates will happily volunteer to serve the community in that capacity. In addition, government should collaborate with corporations to help increase the number and skill level of community public health workers to support the achievement of communities knowledgeable enough to take control of their health.

Obviously, all the recommendations put forth so far, require some level of reading and writing in other to be able to understand the difference between symptoms of disease and witchcraft attacks. In developing countries, a majority of the people still do not know how to read or write. Individuals that lack basic skills in reading and writing are prone to having less exposure to public health education, and little or no developed skills to act on the right information or decision.

As a tool for disease prevention, a literacy campaign is considerably a viable strategy to strengthen our community through research-based knowledge on issues regarding their health. Among other things, strategic collaboration between the government, religious leaders, cooperation and individuals is highly recommended to ensure basic skills in reading and writing are afforded to members of our community. Basic literacy will help them to function effectively in everyday situations, stay updated with new research, discoveries and infection control practices.

Above all, it will help them realize that it is ignoramus not witchcraft!

REFERENCES

About peripheral artery disease (PAD). American Heart Association. http://www.heart.org/HEARTORG/Conditions/More/P eripheralArteryDisease/About-Peripheral-Artery-Disease-PAD_UCM_301301_Article.jsp. Accessed June 20, 2014.

Alternative medicine. Glaucoma Research Foundation. http://www.glaucoma.org/treatment/alternative-medicine.php. Accessed Aug. 2, 2014.

Arrhythmia. National Heart, Lung, and Blood Institute. http://www.nhlbi.nih.gov/health/health-topics/topics/arr/. Accessed July 11, 2014.

August P, et al. Preeclampsia: Clinical features and diagnosis. http://www.uptodate.com/home. Accessed June 7, 2014.

August P. Management of hypertension in pregnant and postpartum women. http://www.uptodate.com/home. Accessed July 4, 2014.

Buhimschi CS, et al. Medications in pregnancy and lactation. Obstetrics and Gynecology. 2009;113:166.

Caplan LR. Etiology and classification of stroke. http://www.uptodate.com/home. Accessed March. 10, 2014.

Caplan LR. Overview of the evaluation of stroke. http://www.uptodate.com/home. Accessed Jan.1 9, 2014.

Cataract causes. American Academy of Ophthalmology. http://www.geteyesmart.org/eyesmart/diseases/cataract s-cause.cfm. Accessed June 2, 2014.

Cataract symptoms. American Academy of Ophthalmology. http://www.geteyesmart.org/eyesmart/diseases/cataract s-symptoms.cfm. Accessed July 2, 2014.

Cataract. American Optometric Association. http://www.aoa.org/cataract.xml. Accessed June 13, 2014.

Cerebral aneurysms fact sheet. National Institute of Neurological Disorders and Stroke. http://www.ninds.nih.gov/disorders/cerebral_aneurysm /cerebral_aneurysms.htm. Accessed June. 19, 2014.

Congenital heart defects. National Heart, Lung, and Blood Institute. http://www.nhlbi.nih.gov/health/health-topics/topics/chd/. Accessed July 1, 2014.

Cooper WO, et al. Major congenital malformations after first-trimester exposure to ACE inhibitors. The New England Journal of Medicine. 2006;354:2443.

Cruz-Knight W, et al. Tuberculosis: An overview. Primary Care Clinics Office Practice. 2013;40:743.

Cucchiara BL, et al. Antiplatelet therapy for secondary prevention of stroke. http://www.uptodate.com/home. Accessed June 2014..

Deak TM, et al. Hypertension and pregnancy. Emergency Medicine Clinics of North America. 2012;30:903.

Diabetes mellitus (DM). The Merck Manuals: The Merck Manual for Health Care Professionals. http://www.merckmanuals.com/professional/endocrine _and_metabolic_disorders/diabetes_mellitus_and_diso rders_of_carbohydrate_metabolism/diabetes_mellitus_ dm.html. Accessed June 10, 2014.

Diarrhea. National Institute for Diabetes and Digestive and Kidney Diseases. http://digestive.niddk.nih.gov/ddiseases/pubs/diarrhea/i ndex.htm. Accessed March 15, 2014.

Diphtheria, tetanus & pertussis vaccines: What you need to know. Centers for Disease Control and Prevention.

http://www.cdc.gov/vaccines/pubs/vis/downloads/vis-dtap.pdf. Accessed March. 15, 2014.

DKA (ketoacidosis) and ketones. American Diabetes Association. http://www.diabetes.org/living-with-diabetes/complications/ketoacidosis-dka.html. Accessed July 9, 2014.

Effects of stroke. National Stroke Association. http://www.stroke.org/site/PageServer?pagename=EFFECT. Accessed Jan. 19, 2014.

Facts about cataract. National Eye Institute. http://www.nei.nih.gov/health/cataract/cataract_facts.asp. Accessed June 12, 2014.

Facts about glaucoma. National Eye Institute. http://www.nei.nih.gov/health/glaucoma/glaucoma_facts.asp. Accessed June 12, 2014.

Furie KL, et al. Etiology and clinical manifestations of transient ischemic attack. http://www.uptodate.com/home. Accessed June 12, 2014.

http://www.accessmedicine.com/resourceTOC.aspx?resourceID=13. Accessed June 12, 2014

Gauer R, et al. Does low-dose aspirin reduce preeclampsia and other maternal-fetal complications? The Journal of Family Practice. 2008;57:54.

Glaucoma risk factors and prevention. National Glaucoma Research. http://www.ahaf.org/glaucoma/about/risk.html. Accessed June 12, 2014.

Glaucoma treatments. National Glaucoma Research. http://www.ahaf.org/glaucoma/treatment/common/. Accessed June 12, 2014.

Glaucoma. American Optometric Association. http://www.aoa.org/Glaucoma.xml. Accessed March 23, 2014.

Go AS, et al. Heart disease and stroke statistics — 2013 update: A report from the American Heart Association. Circulation. 2013;127:e6.

Healthy living with glaucoma. National Glaucoma Research. http://www.ahaf.org/glaucoma/livingwith/healthyliving.html. Accessed July 19, 2014.

High blood pressure and women. American Heart Association. http://www.heart.org/HEARTORG/Conditions/HighBloodPressure/UnderstandYourRiskforHighBloodPressure/High-Blood-Pressure-and-Women_UCM_301867_Article.jsp. Accessed July 7, 2014.

High blood pressure in pregnancy. National Heart, Lung, and Blood Institute. http://www.nhlbi.nih.gov/health/public/heart/hbp/hbp_preg.htm. Accessed July 19, 2014.

Hudelson, P.M., (1993) ORS and Treatment of Childhood Diarrhea in Managua, Nicargua. Journal of Social Science and Medicine; 37(1): 97-103

Hyperglycemia (High blood glucose). American Diabetes Association. http://www.diabetes.org/living-with-diabetes/treatment-and-care/blood-glucose-control/hyperglycemia.html. Accessed July 15, 2014.

Hypertension in pregnancy. The Merck Manual for Health Care Professionals. http://www.merckmanuals.com/professional/sec18/ch261/ch261k.html. Accessed Aug. 1, 2014.

Ischemic stroke (clots). American Stroke Association. http://www.strokeassociation.org/STROKEORG/AboutStroke/TypesofStroke/IschemicClots/Ischemic-Strokes-Clots_UCM_310939_Article.jsp. Accessed June. 9, 2014.

Jacobs DS. Open-angle glaucoma: Epidemiology, clinical presentation, and diagnosis. http://wwwuptodate.com/index. Accessed Aug. 7, 2014.

Jacobs DS. Open-angle glaucoma: Treatment. http://www.uptodate.com/index. Accessed Aug. 2, 2014.

Know stroke brochure. National Institute of Neurological Disorders and Stroke. http://stroke.nih.gov/materials/actintime.htm. Accessed June. 10, 2014.

Low vision resources. Glaucoma Research Foundation. http://www.glaucoma.org/treatment/low-vision-resources.php. Accessed Aug. 2, 2014.

Magloire L, et al. Gestational hypertension. http://www.uptodate.com/home. Accessed June 7, 2014.

Magnani JW, et al. Myocarditis: Current trends in diagnosis and treatment. Circulation. 2006;813:876.

McKulloch DK. Initial management of blood glucose in adults with type 2 diabetes mellitus. http://www.uptodate.com/home. Accessed July 10, 2014.

Medication guide. Glaucoma Research Foundation. http://www.glaucoma.org/treatment/medication-guide.php. Accessed Feb. 26, 2014.

Natural medicines in the clinical management of diabetes. Natural Medicines Comprehensive Database.

http://www.naturaldatabase.com. Accessed June 17, 2014.

Neurological diagnostic tests and procedures. National Institute of Neurological Disorders and Stroke. http://www.ninds.nih.gov/disorders/misc/diagnostic_te sts.htm?css=print. Accessed June 12, 2014

Norwitz ER, et al. Preeclampsia: Management and prognosis. http://www.uptodate.com/home. Accessed June 12, 2014.

Olitsky SE, et al. Overview of glaucoma in infants and children. http://www.uptodate.com/index. Accessed June 12, 2014.

Oliveira-Filho J, et al. Reperfusion therapy for acute ischemic stroke. http://www.uptodate.com/home. Accessed June 12, 2014.

Oliveira-Filho J. Initial assessment and management of acute stroke. http://www.uptodate.com/home. Accessed June 12, 2014.

Preventing eye injuries. American Academy of Ophthalmology. http://www.geteyesmart.org/eyesmart/living/preventin g-eye-injuries.cfm. Accessed March 23, 2014

Prevention and management of wound infection. World Health Organization. http://www.who.int/hac/techguidance/tools/Prevention

%20and%20management%20of%20wound%20infecti
on.pdf. Accessed June 23, 2014.

Questions and answers about carotid endarterectomy.
National Institute of Neurological Disorders and
Stroke.
http://www.ninds.nih.gov/disorders/stroke/carotid_end
arterectomy_backgrounder.htm. Accessed June. 14,
2013.

Questions and answers about tuberculosis. Centers for
Disease Control and Prevention.
http://www.cdc.gov/tb/publications/faqs/default.htm.
Accessed June 17, 2014.

Robertson DM (expert opinion). Mayo Clinic,
Rochester, Minn. Sept. 4, 2012.

Roush SW, et al. Manual for the Surveillance of
Vaccine-Preventable Diseases. 4th ed. Atlanta, Ga.:
Centers for Disease Control and Prevention; 2011.
http://www.cdc.gov/vaccines/pubs/surv-
manual/chpt16-tetanus.html. Accessed June 12, 2014

Samuels OB. Intravenous fibrinolytic (thrombolytic)
therapy in acute ischemic stroke: Therapeutic use.
http://www.uptodate.com/home. Accessed June 12,
2014

Standards of medical care in diabetes — 2014.
Diabetes Care. 2014;37:s14.

Stroke: Hope through research. National Institute of Neurological Disorders and Stroke. http://www.ninds.nih.gov/disorders/stroke/stroke.htm. Accessed June 12, 2014.

Tetanus, diphtheria (Td) or tetanus, diphtheria, pertussis (Tdap) vaccine: What you need to know. Centers for Disease Control and Prevention. http://www.cdc.gov/vaccines/pubs/vis/downloads/vis-td-tdap.pdf. Accessed July 19, 2014.

Tetanus. The Merck Manuals: The Merck Manual for Healthcare Professionals. http://www.merck.com/mmpe/print/sec14/ch178/ch178i.html. Accessed June 13, 2014.

Tetanus: Questions and answers. Immunization Action Coalition. http://www.immunize.org/catg.d/p4220.pdf. Accessed June. 13, 2014.

Vest AR, et al. Hypertension in pregnancy. Cardiology Clinics. 2012;30:407.

Warning signs of a stroke. National Stroke Association. http://www.stroke.org/site/PageServer?pagename=SYMP. Accessed June 19, 2014.

Weizer JS. Angle-closure glaucoma. http://www.uptodate.com/index. Accessed June 77, 2014.

What are cataracts? American Academy of Ophthalmology. http://www.geteyesmart.org/eyesmart/diseases/cataracts.cfm. Accessed July 22, 2014.

What are my options? American Diabetes Association. http://www.diabetes.org/living-with-diabetes/treatment-and-care/medication/oral-medications/what-are-my-options.html. Accessed July 19, 2014.

What are the signs and symptoms of heart disease? National Heart, Lung, and Blood Institute. http://www.nhlbi.nih.gov/health/health-topics/topics/hdw/signs.html. Accessed July 18, 2014.

What is cardiovascular disease? American Heart Association. http://www.heart.org/HEARTORG/Caregiver/Resources/WhatisCardiovascularDisease/What-is-Cardiovascular-Disease_UCM_301852_Article.jsp. Accessed July 23, 2014.

What is the heart? National Heart, Lung, and Blood Institute. http://www.nhlbi.nih.gov/health/health-topics/topics/hhw/. Accessed July 21, 2014.

WHO position paper on Oral Rehydration Salts to reduce mortality from cholera. http://www.who.int/cholera/technical/en/. Accessed August 2, 2014.

Wong EB, et al. Rising to the challenge: new therapies for tuberculosis. Trends in Microbiology. 2013;21:493

Zumla A, et al. Tuberculosis. New England Journal of Medicine. 2013;368:745.

www.ingramcontent.com/pod-product-compliance
Lightning Source LLC
Chambersburg PA
CBHW070659290526
45790CB00001B/385